Terminology for Medical Administrators

MARI ROBBINS
Course Director, Health Studies

JANET WETHERFIELD
Health Studies Lecturer

Foreword by Anthony Yates

Radcliffe Medical Press · Oxford and New York

© 1994 Radcliffe Medical Press Ltd
15 Kings Meadow, Ferry Hinksey Road, Oxford OX2 0DP

Radcliffe Medical Press Inc
141 Fifth Avenue, Suite N, NY 10010, USA

A catalogue record for this book is available from the British Library.

ISBN 1 870905 33 4

Typeset by Acorn Bookwork, Salisbury, Wiltshire
Printed and bound in Great Britain by
Biddles Ltd, Guildford and King's Lynn

Notes for the Reader

The purpose of this book is to shed light on terms and topics that those working in a medical environment are likely to encounter, and perhaps be questioned about by patients. We have *not* attempted to create a comprehensive list of clinical terms, and those seeking to reference the less commonly used terms are advised to consult a conventional medical dictionary. Neither have we sought to give any guidance on diagnosing or treating conditions, and those seeking this information should again consult other sources.

Contents

Foreword   vii

Introduction: Origins of Medical Terminology   1

Structure of the Body and How it Works   3
   Cells and tissues   3
   Body systems   6
   Sensory organs and tissues   17

Definitions   20

Appendix 1: Medical Word Structures   88
              Word roots   89
              Prefixes   93
              Suffixes   96

Appendix 2: Abbreviations and Symbols
              Clinical abbreviations   98
              Other medical abbreviations   106
              Abbreviations used in prescribing   108
              Medical symbols   110

Appendix 3: Immunization Schedules
              Recommended immunizations for children   111
              Recommended immunizations for adults   113

Appendix 4: The Structure of the National Health
              Service   114

Appendix 5: Useful Addresses   116

Foreword

Medicine is one of the oldest professions; in common with law, it tends to complicate or mystify its writings by persistent use of obscure jargon.

Much of medical terminology is derived from Greek, Latin or sometimes hybrid origins. Rationalization will be slow to come and will remain incomplete. An interesting number of lay workers, including administrators, practice managers, medical secretaries, lawyers, social workers and care assistants, are required to be able to interpret medical records, reports and prescriptions.

This new book will be an enormous help to these groups. Having read the text in full, I consider that it will meet the needs of most as a quick, accurate reference source for fundamental anatomical, physiological, clinical and pharmacological terms. The authors, who both have extensive experience of lecturing to health workers, have produced a most valuable basic reference book.

ANTHONY YATES, MD, FRCP
Consultant Rheumatologist
St Thomas's Hospital and King Edward VII Hospital for Officers

Introduction: Origins of Medical Terminology

The early Greeks were the first to develop the distinct role of physician, and it is from their language that many of our current medical terms are derived. Hippocrates, a physician from Kos in Greece about 500 BC, is known as the 'father of medicine'. One of the earliest codes of medical ethics is attributed to him, and still sets standards for doctors today.

With the rise of the Roman Empire, physicians spoke Latin as well as Greek. Hence a further set of medical terms were introduced. The terms have lived on through the centuries, even though the languages in which they were first employed are no longer in daily use.

The word medicine is derived from the Latin **medicina**, which means the science or art of preserving and restoring health. The Greek for 'to heal' is **therapeuein**, from which the words 'therapeutics' and 'therapy' are derived. Terms for modern-day branches of biology and medicine are structured by adapting the Greek word **logos**, meaning 'study of', to '-ology'. 'Neurology', for example, means the study of the nervous system, **neuro** being Greek for 'nerve'.

However, the scientific knowledge and sophisticated equipment which we take for granted in modern medicine did not then exist. Graeco-Roman medicine was based on a system of theoretical beliefs related to the **pneuma** (soul and breath of life), the **psyche** (personification of the soul) and the **soma** (the material body).

Early beliefs also incorporated the 'humoral' theory based on the properties of four bodily fluids, known as **haima** (blood), **phlegma** (phlegm or mucous), **chole** (yellow bile) and **malaina chole** (black bile). The relative proportions of these fluids were thought to determine one's temperament, and disease was attributed to disturbances in the fluid balance: excess of blood caused a sanguine temperament; too much phlegm a cold, unemotional temperament; yellow bile, a hot (choleric) temper; and black bile, ill-humour.

The words associated with these theories, and many others from ancient Greece and Rome, now form the basis of a much more precise and empirical medical language. However, names of physical conditions are still based on those of ancient syndromes: for example, **pneu**monia and **psych**ology. The Latin and Greek word parts listed in Appendix 1 are therefore intended to facilitate understanding of what medical words literally mean, through analysis of their structures.

Structure of the Body and How it Works

The human body may be analysed in terms of its formation –
the materials of which it is constructed – and its functions and
the systems which perform them.

Cells and Tissues

Cells

The body is constructed from billions of cells. Most cells consist
of a fluid called **cytoplasm**, encapsulated in a fine membrane,
and a central nucleus which houses 23 pairs of **chromosomes**
containing genetic material. Cells are capable of performing the
definitive functions of all living matter:

- assimilation of nourishment taken in by the body
- growth and repair (**mitosis**)
- reproduction (**meiosis**)
- excretion of waste products.

Cells are of different types, adapted to specialist functions
according to the tissues to which they belong.

Tissues

There are five main types of tissue:

- **epithelial** – covers the body surface and lines organs and
  cavities

- **connective** – fibrous, areolar, adipose, lymphoid, cartilage and bone
- **muscular** – voluntary, involuntary and cardiac (heart muscle)
- **nervous**
- **blood** – made of **plasma** containing red corpuscles (**erythrocytes**) which carry oxygen to body tissue, white cells (**leucocytes**) which fight infection, and platelets (**thrombocytes**) which help blood to clot to control bleeding.

Red corpuscles contain **haemoglobin**, a pigment which needs iron to maintain its efficiency in attracting oxygen. White cells consist of **phagocytes**, which surround and ingest bacteria, and **lymphocytes** which produce antibodies.

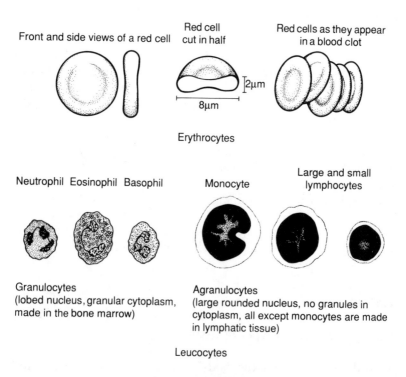

Figure 1 Blood cells

85% of humans are **rhesus positive**; ie they produce **agglutinin** (for immunity) in their red cells. If rhesus positive blood is transfused into a **rhesus negative** recipient, the plasma will produce **agglutinins** (antibodies) which destroy the red cells: hence the need to determine blood groups.

The death of tissue cells **(necrosis)**, from injury or infection, may lead to death of part of the body **(gangrene)**. This is prevented by regeneration by mitosis or by **fibrosis** (ingrowth, causing scarring, in tissue where cells are unable to multiply).

Neoplasms (ie tumours or growths) are clusters of abnormal cells. They grow at the expense of, and imitate, surrounding normal body tissues, and may be **benign** – slow-growing and isolated – or **malignant** – fast growing and tending to spread to other parts of the body.

Body Systems

Tissues and special organs are arranged for working purposes into 'systems' which carry out the functions necessary for the body to remain in health.

The Musculoskeletal System

This is concerned with movement. It consists of bones, muscles, fibrous tissue, ligaments and nerves.

The skeleton

This gives shape and support to the body, anchors muscles, protects internal structures, stores calcium and produces blood cells. A baby is born with 350 bones, but during growth some of these fuse so that the adult human has 206 bones.

Bones can be divided into two main groups: **axial**, consisting of those of the upright parts of the body (skull, vertebrae, ribs and sternum), and **appendicular** (limbs, shoulder girdles and pelvic girdle).

The muscles

Muscles make up the largest mass of tissue in the body and account for approximately 40–50% of body weight. There are more than 600 muscles, which help to move the skeleton and provide strength and warmth.

Involuntary, or smooth, muscles contract automatically and are present in the walls of the major organs. Voluntary muscles are attached to bones; they move the skeletal system and can be controlled at will. Cardiac muscle has a unique structure capable of contracting and relaxing the heart at regular intervals.

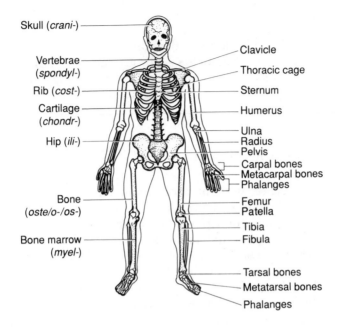

Figure 2 The skeleton

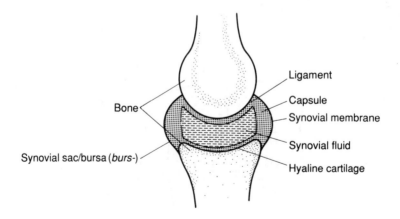

Figure 3 A synovial (freely moveable) joint

Movement

This is articulated by **joints** – the points at which two or more bones join together; **ligaments** – fibrous bands of tissue which connect bones or cartilages and support and strengthen joints; and **tendons** – the fibrous cord by which muscle is attached to bone.

The Respiratory System

This is concerned with breathing and elimination of waste (carbon dioxide and water vapour).

The upper respiratory tract contains the nose and nasal sinuses, the throat (**pharynx**) and voice-box (**larynx**). The lower respiratory tract contains the windpipe (**trachea**), and **bronchi** leading into the **lungs**. The right lung consists of three lobes, but the left lung has only two lobes in order to make way for the heart, which lies in the space between the lungs.

Intercostal muscles and the diaphragm contract and relax in order to enlarge or reduce the size of the **thoracic cavity**, thus sucking air into the lungs or pushing it out.

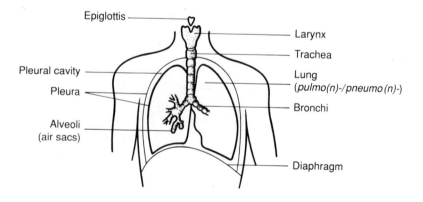

Figure 4 The respiratory system

The Cardiovascular and Circulatory Systems

The heart (**cardiac muscle**) pumps blood around the body via the circulatory system, which is a network of blood vessels. Some of these vessels – the **aorta**, **arteries**, **arterioles** and **capillaries** – carry the blood containing oxygen and nourishment from the heart to the body tissues. Others, consisting of **capillaries**, **venules** and **veins**, return deoxygenated blood and water vapour from the tissues to the heart. The heart relaxes and contracts at an average rate of 70–80 times per minute, and each heartbeat pumps 2 oz of blood into the circulatory system.

The period during which the heart contracts is called **systole** and the relaxation period between contractions, **diastole.** The

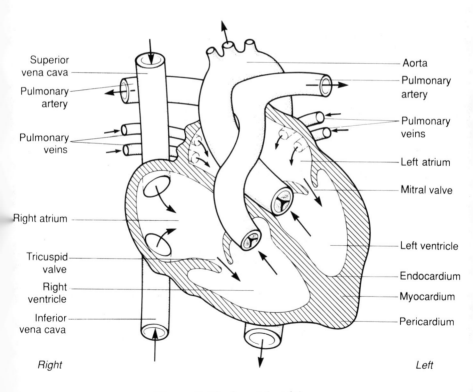

Figure 5 The heart (*cardi-*)

pressure maintained in the circulation by the heart's pumping action is referred to as **blood pressure** and is normally about 40–60 millimetres of mercury higher in systole than diastole. The **pulse** is the impulse felt through the arteries from the heart's contractions, and the sounds we hear when listening to the heartbeat are made by the opening and closing of its valves.

The Digestive System

This system breaks food down, by **mastication** (chewing) and **enzymes** (chemicals), and passes it along the digestive tract and

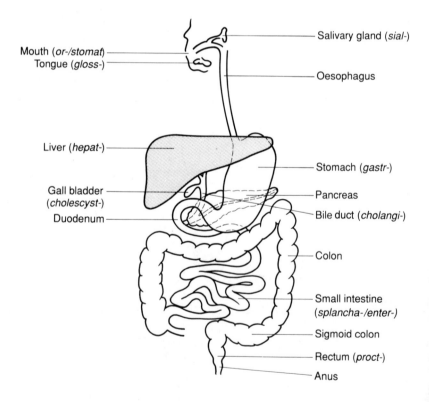

Figure 6 The digestive system

into the bloodstream for storage or energy use, or eliminates it as waste.

Food passes (by means of peristalsis – see page 67) from the mouth to the **pharynx** (throat), into the **oesophagus**, down to the **stomach** and into the **small intestine**, from whence nutrients are absorbed into the bloodstream. The excess passes into the **colon**, where water is absorbed, and then to the **rectum** for storage pending expulsion via the anus.

The Urinary System

The **kidneys** secrete between three and four pints of urine every 24 hours. This is carried by the **ureters** to the **bladder** for storage pending urination through the **urethra** passage.

The urinary system is necessary to excrete waste products, and maintain a normal balance of water, ions (**electrolytes**) and acids in the blood and tissue fluids.

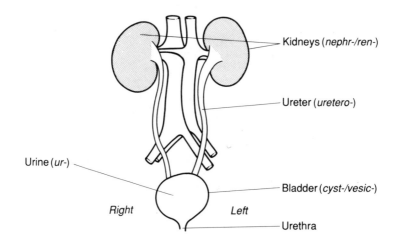

Figure 7 The urinary system

The Reproductive Systems

Male

The internal organs consist of:

- two **testes** – producing **spermatozoa** (male reproductive cells) and **testosterone** (male sex hormone) – and **epididymides** (where sperm are temporarily stored), all contained within the **scrotum**
- the **vas deferens** and **seminal vesicles**
- the **prostate gland.**

The external organ is the **penis** (passage for urine and semen via the **urethra**), which ends in the **glans penis** protected by the foreskin (**prepuce**).

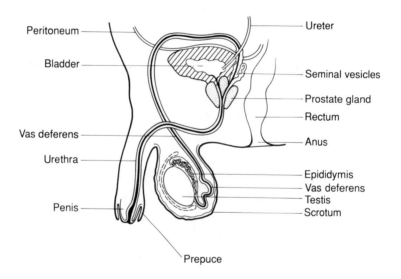

Figure 8 Male reproductive system

Female

From **puberty** to the **menopause**, **ovulation** occurs every 28 days. A mature **ovum** is expelled from one of two **ovaries** (also producing **oestrogen** and **progesterone**, the female sex hormones) and travels along the **uterine tube** to the **uterus** (womb) where (a) it is fertilized by a **spermatozoon** resulting in pregnancy, or (b) it is not fertilized, and **menstruation** occurs.

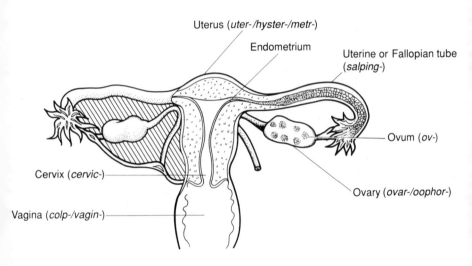

Figure 9 Female reproductive system

If pregnancy occurs, the sperm cell and ovum are united in the uterus within a small membranous bag called the **amniotic sac**. The **embryo** (fertilized ovum) grows in amniotic fluid, and is given sustenance and a blood supply from its mother by the **placenta** (a mass attached to the uterine wall) via the **umbilical cord**.

The Lymphatic System

Lymph is a fluid drained from tissues and incorporating lymphocytes formed in the **lymph glands**, situated throughout the body. It is subsequently collected in the **thoracic and right lymphatic ducts**, and returned to the circulation via lymphatic vessels. The main purpose of this is to fight infection. Lymph glands both destroy bacteria and produce antibodies against those which have survived.

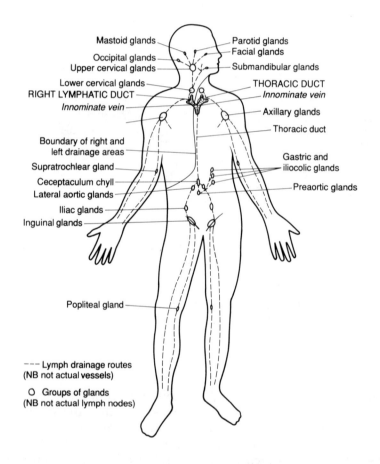

Figure 10 The lymphatic system

The Endocrine System

This is a system of **hormone** production and secretion directly into the bloodstream from specialized **glands**. The affective glands are the **pituitary, thyroid, parathyroid, adrenal, thymus** and **pineal** glands, which are concerned mainly with stimulating and regulating growth, **metabolism** and sexual functions. In addition, the pancreas secretes **insulin** to control carbohydrate metabolism and the gonads (testes and ovaries) secrete sex hormones.

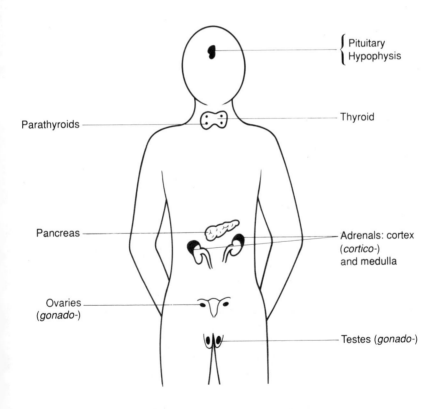

Figure 11 Endocrine glands

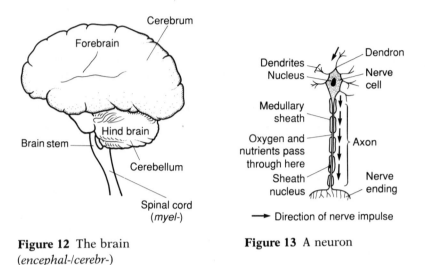

Figure 12 The brain
(*encephal-/cerebr-*)

Figure 13 A neuron

The Nervous System

This is a complex system which carries stimuli between the brain and other body parts. It controls consciousness and mental processes and regulates bodily movements and functions through the dispatch of nerve impulses via nerve cells called **neurons**.

The **central nervous system** consists of the **brain** and **spinal cord**, made of neurons and fibres which convey messages to and from the brain. The **cerebellum** in the brain controls the coordination of muscular activity (via signals transmitted throughout the body by **peripheral nerves**), the **cerebrum** controls all conscious acts and the **brain stem** controls respiration, blood pressure and the heartbeat.

The **autonomic nervous system** comprises nerves that control unconscious acts, ie **parasympathetic nerves** that control the workings of the major organs (eg the heart rate and emptying of the bladder), and **sympathetic nerves** that prepare the body for crises (raise blood pressure and respiration rate, stimulate hormone release and dilate pupils).

Sensory Organs and Tissues

The Eyes

These are made up of three layers:

- the outer supporting fibres called the **sclera**, including the transparent **cornea** over the front of the eye
- the pigmented **choroid coat**, including the **ciliary body** whose muscle controls the amount of light entering the **pupil** and the **iris** which gives the eye its colour
- the inner **retina** from which the optic nerve transmits visual stimuli to the brain.

The bi-concave **lens** lies behind the pupil. It flattens or thickens itself to adjust focus on near or far objects, with the aid of the **suspensory ligaments** to which it is attached. The back chamber inside the eye is filled with **vitreous humour**, a jelly-like fluid which maintains the shape of the eyeball.

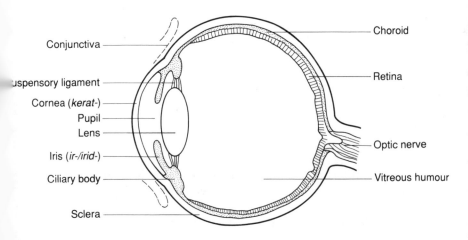

Figure 14 The eye (*ophthalmo-/oculo-*)

The Ears

Sound waves are conveyed from the external ear to the drum, the **tympanic membrane**, at the entrance to the middle ear. Three small bones, the **auditory ossicles**, are arranged to transmit vibrations from the drum to the **oval window** and thence to the inner ear, where balance and hearing are interpreted via the **auditory nerve** to the brain.

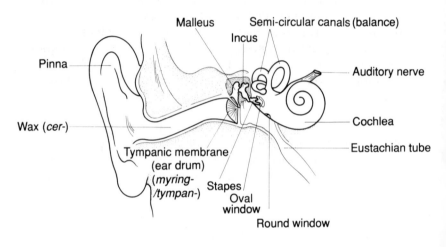

Figure 15 The ear

The Skin

Nerve endings create the sense of touch via the skin, which also protects underlying tissues against pressure and pain, and regulates body temperature. The skin consists of:

- the **epidermis**, made up of dead cells on the surface, and **basal cells** which can reproduce and contain **melanocytes** which produce the pigment **melanin**

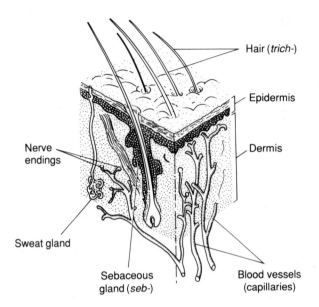

Figure 16 The skin (*derm(at)-/cut-/pell-*)

- the **dermis** beneath, made up of dense connective tissue, hair follicles, nerve endings, blood and lymph vesels, sweat glands and ducts, and sebaceous glands for lubrication
- **subcutaneous tissue** ('under the skin') containing fatty deposits.

Definitions

abdomen the lower trunk or the largest body cavity (hollow), which is situated in the trunk, immediately below the thorax from which it is separated by the diaphragm; houses the digestive organs, most of the glands and the kidneys; term may also include the pelvic cavity beneath, which houses the female reproductive organs, bladder and bowels

abscess a localized collection of pus, eg a boil, created by germs gaining access to the tissue from an injury or disease in a neighbouring organ; may produce heat, swelling and pain, and eventually burst; treated by lancing or with antibiotics

accommodation the eye's ability to adjust the convexity of its lense to focus clearly on different distances

acne vulgaris (acne) inflammation of the sebaceous (sweat) glands, caused by overstimulation, often when hormones are imbalanced during adolesence, and resulting in pimples and blackheads when pores become blocked

acquired a long-term condition or disease that is 'caught' as opposed to having been present at birth; *cf* **hereditory** and **congenital**

acquired immune deficiency syndrome *see* **AIDS**

acupuncture Chinese technique for relieving pain, treating disease or producing anaesthesia, by inserting special needles into particular parts of the body

acute adjective indicating rapid onset and short duration of disease, not necessarily indicating severity; *cf* **chronic**

Addison's disease condition characterized by weakness, weight loss, poor appetite, low blood pressure and skin pigmentation, and caused by deficient secretion of hormones from the adrenal glands

adenoids pads of lymphoid tissue in the upper throat beside the tonsils, both of which aid bacterial immunity and shrink during adoescence; or enlargement of adenoids caused by infection, which may cause nasal obstruction and interfere with hearing

adhesion abnormal union of fibrous tissues which should be freely moveable, often following inflammation after injury or abdominal surgery

adipose tissue (fatty tissue) type of connective tissue made of fat globules and membranes

adrenal glands situated above each kidney, and consisting of the outer cortex, which secretes hormones affecting metabolism and aiding development of secondary sexual characteristics, and the inner medulla, which secretes the hormones adrenalin and noradrenalin

adrenalin hormone secreted from the medulla of the adrenal glands as a response to fear, and which prepares the body to fight or flee by raising blood pressure, mobilizing energy and dilating bronchial vessels to allow greater use of oxygen; may be manufactured synthetically to treat asthma or circulatory problems

afterbirth the placenta, cord and membranes which are expelled from the uterus after childbirth

agglutinogen a substance produced in the red blood cells of 85% of humans (rhesus positive). **agglutinin** an antibody formed in the red blood cells of rhesus negative people against agglutinogen introduced into their circulation in blood from an incompatible group. **agglutination** the clumping of red blood cells caused by agglutinins

AIDS (acquired immune deficiency syndrome) a syndrome that damages the immune system, so that the sufferer loses his or her ability to overcome disease or infection; caused by a virus (HIV) which enters the bloodstream via infected body fluids of another person; may have an incubation period of several years before any symptoms present; *see also* **HIV positive**

alimentary canal collective term for the route which food takes from the mouth to the large intestine through the organs of digestion

allergic rhinitis (hayfever) an allergy to pollen which, in certain summer conditions, causes cold-like symptoms and sometimes difficulty in breathing

alopecia (baldness) common, usually congenital, condition among adult males. **alopecia areata** patchy hair loss, often in children, brought on by physical or emotional trauma

alternative medicine *see* **complementary medicine**

amenorrhoea absence of menstruation; may be primary, when menstruation fails to commence at puberty, or secondary, when menstruation ceases prematurely

amnesia complete loss of memory in respect of a period of time; may result from concussion or dementia

amniocentesis removal in the 14th week of pregnancy of a sample of amniotic fluid surrounding the growing fetus, for examination to detect any congenital abnormalities (eg spina bifida); usually offered to women in high risk groups

amphetamine a chemical stimulant, formerly prescribed as an appetite depressant or to treat depression, but whose use is now restricted due to its addictive potential and frequent abuse

anaemia deficiency of haemoglobin (which circulates oxygen around the body and contains iron) in the blood due to lack of red blood cells and/or their haemoglobin content; often caused by lack of iron in the diet and may result in skin pallor, tiredness and breathlessness. **pernicious anaemia (PA)** due to deficient absorption of vitamin B_{12} which prevents red blood cell formation in bone marrow. **sickle-cell anaemia** peculiar to black people, and caused by a hereditory abnormality in the haemoglobin; the red blood cells take on a sickle-like shape

anaesthesia loss of sensation. **anaesthetic** drug that induces anaesthesia; may be general, causing loss of consciousness, or local, in which nerve conduction is blocked from a specific area to numb it. **anaesthetist** person qualified to administer anaesthetics

analgesic any pain-relieving drug

angina constricting sensation and pain in the chest caused by inadequate blood supply to the heart muscle, often after exertion

angiogram/angiography X-ray film/recording using contrast dye to detect abnormality or obstruction of a blood or lymph vessel, eg of the cerebral vessels in the brain. **angiocardiography** X-ray of heart structure by injecting radio-opaque dye, to test for cardiac abnormality

anorexia loss of appetite. **anorexia nervosa (AN)** psychological disturbance resulting in loss of appetite, most common in female adolescents. **bulimia** psychological eating disorder characterized by binge and vomit cycles

anterior pertaining to the front surface of the body

antibiotic an antibacterial drug produced from a fungus or another bacterium, eg penicillin, which stimulates production of antibodies

antibody (immunoglobulin) a protein produced in white blood cells, stimulated by a foreign body invader to produce immunity against it. **antigen** substance capable of stimulating antibody production; usually a protein in an invading germ

anticoagulant an agent which reduces the blood's ability to clot, used in some blood or heart conditions or on blood obtained for investigation or transfusion

antihistamine drug used to suppress allergic reactions, eg hayfever, or to relieve motion sickness

antinuclear factor/antibody (ANF/ANA) blood test to diagnose systemic lupus erythematosis (SLE)

antisepsis prevention of tissue infection. **antiseptic** chemical substance which destroys or inhibits growth of organisms liable to cause infection

anuria complete cessation of urine formation by the kidneys

aorta the main artery arising out of the left ventricle of the heart, and part of the network of tubes which carry blood away from the heart and into circulation; *see* Figure 5. **aortogram** an angiogram test for abnormality of the aorta by injection of radio-opaque dye

apical heart rate measurement of the heart's beat at its apex using a stethoscope, to detect irregularity of the pulse

apoplexy *see* **cerebrovascular accident**

appendicular skeleton umbrella term for the 'appendages' to the skeleton, consisting of the limbs, shoulder girdles, and pelvic girdle

appendix small patent tube at the junction between small and large intestines; has no known function. **appendicitis** inflammation of the appendix characterized by severe abdominal pain. **appendicectomy** surgical removal of the appendix

areolar tissue type of 'packing' connective tissue

artery one of a network of vessels which carry blood away from the heart and into circulation; branch into arterioles and capillaries. **pulmonary artery** the primary artery emanating from the heart; *see* Figure 5. **arteriogram** an angiogram (X-ray using radio-opaque dye) of the arteries

arthritis Inflammation of the joints, causing pain and often resulting in deformities of the hands, knees or feet.
oesteoarthritis degenerative arthritis, occurring mainly in middle and old age. **rheumatoid arthritis** inflammation of multiple, usually peripheral joints, and connective tissue, resulting in crippling deformities, muscle wasting and general ill health; *see also* **rheumatism**. **arthrogram** radiographic examination of the internal structure of a joint, to test for an abnormality. **arthroscopy** visual inspection of a joint through a lighted tube (**arthroscope**)

artificial insemination treatment for infertility by instrumental injection of semen into the vagina at time of ovulation

ascitic fluid *see* **paracentesis**

asthma (bronchial asthma) recurring sudden difficulty in breathing due to a muscular spasm in the bronchi which impedes air flow; chronic, often hereditory disease whose attacks may be precipitated by direct irritation, infection, allergy or psychological factors; symptoms treatable by inhaled adrenalin or other drugs

aspiration *see* **paracentesis**

astigmatism blurring or distorted vision when images fail to converge on the retina due to an abnormal curvature of the cornea or lens; may be congenital or acquired

atrophy shrinkage or wastage of tissues or organs; may be local or general; causes include normal ageing, disuse (of limbs), interference with nerve or blood supply, infection or toxins

attached staff members of a primary health care team who work in association with a general practice but who are employed by the District Health Authority rather than by the GP partners; these include district nurses, health visitors, community midwives, social workers and community psychiatric nurses

audiometry hearing assessment. **audiometer** mechanical apparatus used to assess hearing, which generates tones of varying pitch and intensity. **audiometrist** person qualified to carry out audiometry

audit (clinical audit) method used by health professionals to assess the quality of patient care in a systematic way with a view to improvement; involves defining standards, collecting and analysing performance data and identifying changes that may be made

auriscopy visual ear examination using an **auriscope**, a fine flexible tube which transmits light into the ear to permit examination, photography or biopsy; *see also* **endoscopy**

Australia antigen – hepatitis B blood test to diagnose serum hepatitis

autonomic nervous system (ANS) part of the nervous system, which is concerned with reflex control of bodily functions. **sympathetic nerves** nerve types within the ANS which prepare the body for emergencies; they raise blood pressure and flow, dilate bronchi to allow more air into the lungs, postpone digestion and excretion, dilate pupils and raise hairs, and stimulate flow of adrenalin; *cf* **adrenalin**. **parasymaphetic nerves** 'restore peace' by reversing emergency reflexes; *see also* page 16

axial skeleton the bones of the axis of the body: the skull, vertebrae, ribs and sternum

Babinski's sign *see* **plantar reflex**

bacteria single-celled micro-organisms; some strains are parasitic on animals (including humans) or plants, and can cause decomposition or disease (or be beneficial) as they multiply rapidly within the body. **pathogenic bacteria** bacteria associated with specific diseases

barbiturates commonly used group of sedative drugs, employed for short-term general anaesthesia or as a tranquilizer; can have side-effects or become addictive, causing psychological dependence or increasing tolerance resulting in higher dosage and the risk of overdose

barium meal test for lesions (damaged tissue) in the stomach or duodenum; patient drinks solution and films are taken at intervals of its passage into the stomach. **barium swallow** test similar to barium meal for damage to the oesophagus (the gullet), using a visualization technique called fluoroscopy. **barium enema** barium sulphate is administered into the bowel via the rectum, and a fluoroscopy made of bowel movement

Basic Practice Allowance payment made by the Family Health Services Authority to all full-time GPs, dependent on a minimum list size; this is the foundation of a GP's income, intended to cover practice expenditure, and which is supplemented by capitation fees (page 30) and item-of-service payments (page 54)

benign harmless or not serious; usually refers to a non-cancerous tumour

Better Living, Better Life a Department of Health publication (1993) which issues guidelines on health promotion (*see* page 49) and advocates techniques for effective patient counselling for a healthier lifestyle; covers such topics as screening, diet and cholesterol, smoking, etc

bile green-yellow fluid secreted by the liver and stored in the gall-bladder; used in the digestion of fats

biliary colic cramp-like pain caused by 'stones' entering the common bile duct from the gall-bladder

bilious in correct usage vomit containing bile, or vomiting and discomfort caused by acute indigestion

biochemistry the study of the chemistry of living things

biopsy the surgical removal of a piece of tissue for examination (for infection or malignancy), performed under either local or general aesthetic

bladder membranous sac containing fluid or gas. **urinary bladder** expanding sac made of involuntary muscle and used to store urine which is carried to it from the kidneys; *see also* page 11. **gall-bladder** pear-shaped muscular bag on the under-surface of the liver which stores bile, a fluid aiding digestion. **gallstones** 'stones' formed in the gall-bladder, which may be multi-faceted and are composed of bile pigment, calcium or cholesterol

blood groups blood classification based on the ABO system, wherein the groups A, B, and AB contain corresponding antigens and O contains none; receipt of mismatching antigens through transfusion causes agglutination (AB people are 'universal recipients' and O people 'universal donors'). In addition, everyone is either rhesus positive or negative, and these cannot be mixed either; *see also* page 5 and **agglutinogen**

blood pressure (BP) the pressure maintained in the arteries by the heart's pumping action, measured in millimetres of mercury as the heart contracts (systole) and relaxes (diastole); *see also* page 10. **sphygomanometer** instrument used to measure BP by means of an inflatable cuff which is wrapped around the patient's arm

blood urea test to find out how much urea (end-product of protein metabolism) is in the blood; indicator, if raised, of kidney disease

bone connective tissue consisting of a hard dense shell (**compact bone**) made of calcium deposits and inside a porous substance (**cancellous bone**) which supports blood vessels and bone marrow. **bone marrow** a substance contained in the bone cavities, which in early life promotes blood formation

bone scan injection of radio-isotopes to detect secondary tumours and other diseases

bradycardia an abnormally slow pulse rate

brain stem part of the central nervous system, located within the cranium; *see* page 16

breech presentation 'upside down' position of child in the womb, so that it will be born buttocks rather than head first

British Medical Association (BMA) the largest medical association in the UK, which is concerned with nearly every aspect of medicine and medical affairs, and is recognized as one of the principal bodies representing British doctors; incorporates the **General Consultants' and Specialists' Committee** (page 45) and the **General Medical Services Committee** (page 45)

British National Formulary (BNF) annual publication, issued free to all doctors, that lists all drugs by their generic (*see* page 46) and proprietary names

bronchi two tubes into which the trachea (windpipe) divides at its lower end. **bronchioles** sub-divisions of the bronchi which terminate in air sacs (alveoli) in the lungs; *see* Figure 4. **bronchitis** short or long-term inflammation of the bronchi; can occur as a complication of common infectious childhood diseases, or chronically, often due to smoking, when symptoms are a productive cough or breathing difficulty

bronchoscopy visual examination of the interior of the bronchi by means of a thin telescopic instrument passed through the windpipe; used to detect inhaled foreign objects or to diagnose lung diseases. **bronchoscope** instrument used to perform bronchoscopy. **bronchography** X-ray to diagnose bronchial abnormalities

bullae large watery blisters characteristic of some skin diseases

bursitis inflammation of the 'cushion' (bursa) protecting a joint, commonly occurring in the elbow or knee

bypass surgery heart surgery which involves bypassing diseased segments of the arteries (enabling free circulation) by venous grafts, usually undertaken to relieve angina

cadaver a dead body which is dissected in medical school or in a mortuary at a post-mortem

caesarean section delivery of the fetus through surgical incision through the walls of the abdomen and uterus; said to be named after Caesar, who is alleged to have been born this way

calcification hardening of tissues due to deposits of calcium salts within them; normal in growth and development of bones and teeth, but can occur pathologically in joints or arteries

cancer general term desribing a parasitic malignant growth of useless tissue, which disrupts the function of a part of the body and may spread to other areas. There are three types: **carcinoma** affecting the cells on the body surface and which line organs and cavities (epithelial); **sarcoma** affecting connective tissue cells; and **leukaemia** affecting white blood cells

Candida yeast-like fungus which causes oral and genital infections (eg thrush); most susceptible are those with weakened immunity due to existing pathology

capitation fees standard payments made to GPs for each patient registered on their lists, now expected to account for about 60% of GPs' NHS remuneration. There are increments for patients at 65 and 75 years old to reflect additional workload associated with older patients

carbuncle acute inflammation of subcutaneous skin tissue, with discharges and sloughing of tissue (shedding of dead cells), usually caused by the bacterium *Staphylococcus*

carcinoma *see* **cancer**

cardiac pertaining to the heart. **cardiac arrest** complete cessation of the heart's activity

cardiology study of the heart. **cardiologist** heart specialist

cardiovascular system (CVS) body system consisting of the heart, arteries and veins; *see* page 9.

carpal bones wrist bones; *see also* **metacarpals** and **phalanges**. **carpal tunnel syndrome** pain caused by pressure of the inflamed median nerve in the wrist and hand; common during pregancy, and for those suffering forms of arthritis and diabetes

cartilage a dense connective tissue in the joints, discs between vertebrae, ribs, larynx, trachea, ears and nose; capable of withstanding pressure; some is elastine for flexibility

casualty person injured in accident or war

casualty department part of a hospital where casualties are treated, now more commonly known as an accident and emergency department

cataract partial or complete opacity of the lens in the eye, causing blurring of sight and eventually blindness; may be senile, congenital, traumatic or associated with diabetes, and is operable

catarrh excessive secretions from the mucous lining of the nose and throat, commonly associated with a cold or chronically with enlarged adenoids

catheterization the passing of a **catheter** (small tube) into the body, usually into the bladder for urine drainage in cases of retention; or into the heart via the veins for pressure measurement and to take blood samples

catheter specimen of urine (CSU) sterile sample obtained to test for excess of a substance which might indicate disease: tests are Albustix or Utristix for protein, Clinitest for sugar, Haemastix for blood, and Labstix or Multistix for various substances. **midstream specimen of urine (MSU)** specimen of urine obtained from midstream

cellulite lumping of fatty tissue causing puckering of the skin, especially on women's hips and thighs. **cellulitis** inflammation of subutaneous tissue (under the skin surface)

central nervous system (CNS) the brain and spinal cord; *see* page 16

central venous pressure measurement of blood pressure in the superior vena cava (vein entering the heart), via a catheter introduced into a vein in the arm and passed through the system of veins; low pressure may result from dehydration or haemorrhage, and high pressure from heart failure

cerebellum the part of the brain that controls the co-ordination of muscle activity; *see* page 16

cerebral palsy congenital, non-progressive brain damage resulting in varying degrees of spasticity (paralysis, spasms or inability to control muscles in the limbs)

cerebrovascular accident (apoplexy, stroke) interference with blood flow into the brain; extent of damage varies, may result in local paralysis depending on site in the brain affected. Causes are: **haemorrhage** bursting of small blood vessel in the brain; **embolism** blocking of a blood vessel by a fatty deposit or air; **thrombosis** blocking of a vessel by a blood clot

cerebrum the part of the brain that controls conscious acts; *see* page 16

cervical cytology (smear) removal of cells from the cervix (neck of the womb) to detect abnormal (pre-cancerous) cells and other conditions; test generally performed every three years on sexually active women

cervix neck of an organ, especially the uterus (womb)

chemotherapy (CT) use of a chemical agent introduced into the blood to arrest progress of or eradicate disease without damaging healthy tissue

chicken pox *see* **varicella**

child health surveillance programme of preventive care and health promotion provided by GPs (for a special fee since the 1990 Contract), paediatricians, health visitors and nurses

chilblains (erythema pernio) inflammation of the skin, with itching and burning sensation in exposed parts of the hands and feet and tip of the nose; cellular damage as reaction to cold due to local circulatory deficiency

chiropody professional maintenance of feet and treatment of minor foot disorders. **chiropodist** person practising chiropody

chiropractic manipulation of the vertebrae to treat mechanical disorders, based on theory of releasing trapped nerves. **chiropractor** person (not a doctor) who performs chiropractic techniques

cholecystectomy surgical removal of the gall-bladder (*see* **bladder**); usually advised in cases of stones or inflammation. **cholecystography** test for gallstones, by means of X-rays before and after food, after swallowing of an opaque substance

cholesterol crystalline fatty substance found in the brain, nerves, blood and bile; important in metabolism; individuals have varying amounts and diet also affects its formation, high levels being a contributary cause of heart disease

chromosome rod-shaped genetic carrier which contain genes, the determinants of hereditory characteristics; 23 pairs are situated in the nucleus of every human cell except in the mature ovum and sperm; in women including one pair of x chromosomes and in men one x and one y chromosome, whose combination determines the sex of offspring

chronic adjective indicating longstanding disease or condition, regardless of degree of severity; *cf* **acute**

cineradiograph a moving picture X-ray, taken to watch functioning of a joint, tendon or organ

circumcision excision or part excision of prepuce (foreskin) of the penis; at birth or puberty to prevent tightening or as a religious or cultural rite. **female circumcision** excision of the clitoris and (sometimes) suturing of the vulval lips to prevent intercourse

cirrhosis hardening of an organ. **cirrhosis of liver** progressive chronic destruction of liver tissues leading to impaired function or jaundice; may result from dietary deficiency or, most often, from alcoholism

cisternal puncture *see* **lumbar puncture**

clavicle (collar-bone) part of the shoulder girdle in the skeleton

cleft lip/palate congenital incomplete fusion of upper lip and palate

clonus response test which attempts to stimulate muscle contractions, eg in the ankle, to detect disease of the central nervous system

clotting time length of time taken for blood to clot, normally 4–7 minutes; laboratory test may be carried out if patient suspected of having haemophilia, jaundice, or other disease which slows clotting time

coccyx last four bones fused at the base of the vertebral column

coitus the act of sexual intercourse

colic severe pain resulting from periodic spasms in the abdomen; various causes. **biliary colic** *see* **bile**

collagen tough white protein, the main constituent of tissue in the tendons and joint capsules; inflammatory and other conditions can result from collagen malfunction

colon the large intestine (large bowel) into which unabsorbed food passes and is drained to leave faeces. **colonoscopy** inspection of colon by means of a colonoscope, a specialized endoscope (page 41), to detect a tumour or disease

colour blindness inability to distinguish between certain colours, commonly red and green; more prevalent among men than women

coma an unconscious state from which a person cannot be roused and is unresponsive to stimuli; can occur as a result of very serious illness, severe intoxication or head injury

comedones blackheads

community care care of the old or the mentally or physically disabled in their homes, with the aid of local health and social services, as opposed to in hospital or a residential institution. It is currently Government policy as far as possible to integrate the mentally ill into the community, rather than care for them in institutions

Community Health Council (CHC) statutory body set up by the Regional Health Authority to represent the public interest in the local provision of health services, and as a channel for consumer concerns; generally one per District Health Authority

complementary medicine (alternative medicine) methods of medicinal treatment supported by a different philosophical/knowledge base to conventional therapies offered by doctors; many forms originate with non-Western societies; now often used in conjunction with conventional treatments

compression damage to the brain due to pressure from the skull

concussion 'shaking up' of brain tissue, as a result of a blow or fall, which may result in loss of consciousness for a short time, a dazed feeling or disorientation

congenital abnormal condition present at birth which may be hereditory (due to genetic factors) or resulting from unfavourable conditions in the womb or during delivery

conjunctivitis inflammation of the conjunctiva (membrane covering the front of the eye) usually due to environmental irritation

consultant a doctor who is qualified in a medical specialty, eg a consultant cardiologist; may be a senior hospital doctor or run a private clinic; GPs refer patients to appropriate consultants in cases of serious illness or if they are unable to make a diagnosis or initiate care themselves

contraception prevention of conception; artificial methods include (a) mechanical means – condom, cervical cap or intrauterine device (implanted in the womb) – or (b) oral contraception (pills containing female hormones which prevent release of the ovum)

contusion bleeding in the subcutaneous layer of the skin (bruise)

convulsions (fits) involuntary muscle contractions; may be caused by temporary or permanent brain damage or occur during a fever (especially in children); severe fits may be accompanied by loss of consciousness; *see* **epilepsy**

Coombs' test test for antibodies coating red blood cells, which are deficient in babies with haemolytic disease of the newborn (due to Rhesus incompatibility with the mother)

cornea transparent curved membrane in the front of the eye, which covers the iris and pupil. **corneal reflex** method of acertaining degree of unconsciousness or anaesthesia, by whether eyes automatically close in response to touching of the conjunctivae

coronary pertaining to vessels that serve the heart. **coronary thrombosis** a heart attack caused by blocking of a coronary artery with a thrombus (clot)

cortisone an anti-stress hormone secreted by the adrenal glands above the kidneys

cost-rent scheme NHS initiative offering financial incentives for GP partnerships to build or convert premises, or to improve existing premises. The scheme was introduced in the 1970s with the aim of covering the interest on project loans, and revised in the 1990 Contract which introduced a cash limit dependent on local availability

cranium the part of the skull enclosing the brain

creatinine clearance test laboratory test of blood and urine to detect impairment of kidney function. **urea clearance test** laboratory test of blood and urine indicates extent of confirmed kidney damage

cretinism congenital physical and mental underdevelopment resulting from a thyroid gland deficiency (*see* page 81); characterized by stunted growth with large tongue, pot belly and clumsy gait

cyanosis a blue tinge to the skin, lips and tongue which indicates that the blood circulating in the body is lacking in oxygen

cystitis inflammation of the urinary bladder caused by an infection, which affects mainly women and results in urine being passed frequently and painfully. **cystogram** X-ray of the urinary bladder as it fills, to detect disease. **cystoscopy** visual inspection (through a cystoscope) of the urinary bladder, to detect disease or obtain tissue for biopsy, or for diathermy

cytology the study of the body's cells; *see* page 3

cytoplasm fluid of which most of every cell is formed

cytotoxics (literally substances poisonous to cells) drugs used to treat malignant cells, eg in tumours

degenerative of chronic disease or condition that worsens as time goes by; the deterioration is usually irreversible

dementia irreversible brain disease causing disorientation and loss of memory and ability to reason; usually occurring in old age (senile dementia)

dermatitis inflammation of the skin with reddening, blistering and itchiness; frequently due to contact with a substance to which person is allergic

dermatology study of the skin and abnormal skin conditions

dermis the layer of the skin under the epidermis, which contains hair follicles, nerve endings, blood and lymph vessels, and sweat glands

detached retina separation of the inner tissue of the eye (retina) from the middle layer (choroid coat) as a result of trauma (a 'knocking') or disease; *see* page 17

diabetes mellitus disorder of the glands in the pancreas which produce insulin. Insulin is necessary for extracting energy from carbohydtrates (metabolism). Diabetics produce too little insulin which results in a build-up of sugar (a type of carbohydrate) in the blood, and this must be compensated for by a low carbohydrate diet and/or taking of pills containing insulin (for non-insulin dependent diabetics (NIDDs), usually those who develop the disease in later life) or by daily insulin injections (for insulin dependent diabetics (IDDs), who usually develop the disease in childhood)

diagnosis identification of a disease from a patient's symptoms; *cf* **prognosis**

Dick test test in which a small quantity of scarlet fever bacteria are injected into the skin, to ascertain susceptibility to the disease

differential agglutination test (DAT) test for rheumatoid arthritis, which proves positive if sheep serum agglutinates patient's blood sample

differential white blood count test to ascertain the proportion of different white cells in various diseases

digestive enzymes chemicals secreted in the digestive organs which act as catalysts (speeding agents) in the process of breaking down and altering the structure of food particles

digestive system network of organs that perform a series of steps to convert food into a state capable of being stored by the body for energy and tissue nourishment; *see* page 11

dilatation and curettage (D & C) surgical widening of the cervix and removal of specimen tissue from the womb for analysis; may be carried out to investigate excessively heavy periods or a suspected hormone imbalance or tumour

diphtheria an infectious disease in which an inflammed discharge forms in the throat; once common and often fatal, but now children are immunized against it

diplopia double vision caused by each eye forming a separate image on its retina and failure of the eye muscles to bring these images together

dispensing practice a general practice authorized to issue medicines directly to patients rather than give them presciptions for the local pharmacist to supply; often applies to practices in remote rural areas

District Health Authority (DHA) these are the next tier down (from central to local management in the NHS) from Regional Health Authorities; responsible for purchasing hospital and community services for residents in a given area – there are 197 in England and Wales

district/community nurse a nurse who is employed by the District Health Authority to visit ill people in their homes; may be 'attached' to a general practice (page 26)

diuretic drug which drains excess fluid from the tissues and consequently increases the quantity of urine excreted by the kidneys; given to patients who have an accumulation of fluid in their body tissues due to longstanding heart or kidney disease

domiciliary visit/care home visit to a patient by a doctor, district nurse or other health worker; or care in a nursing home

dorsal biological term referring to the back surface of the body; *cf* **ventral**

Down's syndrome a congenital (present at birth) brain disorder resulting in severe mental retardation; the adult sufferer normally has a mental age of less than eight years old

dwarfism underdevelopment of body; achondroplastic dwarves have a relatively large head and short extremities

dysentery bacterial infection causing inflammation of the large intestine (colon), often accompanied by ulcers, and always by severe diarrhoea and abdominal pain; common in the tropics when water or food becomes contaminated

dyslexia inability to read properly due to a brain disorder which causes letters to become confused or their order in a word altered; does not affect normal intelligence

dysmenorrhoea painful menstruation

dyspepsia indigestion

dyspnoea   difficulty in breathing

echocardiography test using an ultrasound beam, to detect disease of the heart's valves or escape of fluid into the area surrounding the heart

ectopic pregnancy development of the embryo outside the womb, usually in the wall of one of the Fallopian tubes (*see* page 43), causing bleeding and pain; the embryo must be surgically removed to avert danger to the mother

eczema skin inflammation and itching, sometimes with blistering, caused by a chemical irritant or allergy

elastin yellow protein with elastic property, present in ligaments and arteries to enable stretching

electrocardiogram (ECG) procedure which uses a special machine to measure the electrical charges in the heart; the machine (**electrocardiograph**) produces a record of the heart's impulses as a tracing on paper, which reveals any disturbances to the normal rythmn; sometimes carried out by the GP

electroencephalogram (EEG) recording of the electrical activity of the brain, to locate swellings or find the cause of fits

electromyogram (EMG) recording of the electrical activity of a muscle: abnormal patterns indicate disease

embryo the fertilized ovum (egg) which grows in the womb of the mother; it divides into multiple cells and forms a placenta which collects sustenance from the mother and passes it on through the umbilical cord; after two months, when it becomes recogizably human, the developing child becomes known as the fetus

encephalogram test for brain tumours, involving lumbar puncture (to free cerebrospinal fluid) and injection of air into the void

enema administration of a liquid into the rectum, eg to expel faeces, for nourishment, sedative effect or X-ray diagnosis

endemic *see* **epidemiology**

endocrine system collection of glands, distributed around the body, whose purpose is to secrete hormones directly into the bloodstream, to assist in various bodily functions; *see* page 15

endometriosis the presence of specialized cells outside their normal site in the lining of the womb (**endometrium**); the cells cause bleeding and pain

endoscopic retrograde cholangio-pancreatography (ERCP) X-ray, involving a specialized endoscope, of the biliary tract; to detect tumours in the tract or cancer of the pancreas

endoscopy investigative procedure used to look at or take samples from internal organs; carried out by means of a flexible lighted tube (**endoscope**) passed into the body through an orifice or small incision

enzyme *see* **digestive enzyme**

epidemic/infectious parotitis (mumps) acute infectious disease caused by a virus and resulting in inflammation of the parotid glands beneath the ears; common in childhood

epidemiology the science that studies diseases in the community: their prevalence, who is affected, how the diseases are spread and their effects. **epidemic** an outbreak of a disease similtaneously affecting a large number of people. **endemic** persistant high incidence of a disease in a community

epidermis protective outer layer of the skin made of dead cells without a blood supply

epididymis part of the male genitalia: a temporary storage site for sperm

epiglottis flap of cartilage at the back of the throat, which presses against the opening of the voice box during swallowing to prevent food from going down the trachea (windpipe)

epilepsy brain disorder that periodically causes a sudden momentary or longer loss of consciousness, which in more serious cases is preceded by convulsions and muscular rigidity (an epileptic fit)

epithelium type of cell that covers the surface of the skin and lines organs and cavities

eruption a rash

erythema reddening of the skin which usually indicates either the onset of a fever or an allergy

erythrocytes *see* **red blood corpuscles**

erythrocyte sedimentation rate (ESR) (Westergren or Wintrobe) measurement of the settling of a sample of red blood cells in a test tube; used to detect or view progress of various diseases of body systems

ethics code of professional conduct to guide doctors and other health workers in their behaviour towards patients; based on the Hippocratic Oath drawn up by Hippocrates in the fourth centry BC, and reformulated for modern application in the Declaration of Geneva issued by the World Health Organization in 1941

excision surgical removal of internal tissue or an organ

excercise tolerance test taking of the pulse before and after specific excercises to estimate the patient's reserve of endurance in case of heart disease

exfoliation 1. excessive loss of surface layers of the skin in thin flakes, symptomatic of a skin disorder 2. the shedding of 'milk' teeth

faeces *see* **stools**

Fallopian tubes (uterine tubes) two tubes in the woman's reproductive system, that transport eggs (ova) from the ovaries to the womb (uterus); *see* page 13

Family Health Services Authority (FHSA) managing body.in a given area (often the same as that of the District Health Authority) for the services provided by general medical practitioners, general dental practitioners, pharmacists and opticians, who are all independent contractors (*not* employees of the NHS) (*see* page 45); there are 90 FHSAs in England and Wales

febrile convulsion fit brought on by fever which can affect children aged four to six years old

femur the thigh bone, which is the longest and strongest bone in the body

fetus/foetus the developing child in its mother's womb; term used from the beginning of the third month following implantation, as this is when it becomes recognizably human; *see also* **embryo**

fibula the thin outer bone running the length of the calf; *see* Figure 2

fluoroscopy method of looking at internal organs wherein the organ and its functional movement is visualized on a fluorescent screen

foetus *see* **fetus**

forced expiratory volume (FEV) the maximum amount of air that can be forcibly breathed out in one second; if low may indicate lung disease

forceps delivery childbirth aided by grasping and pulling the baby's skull with a specialized instrument

fundholding pertaining to a general medical practice which holds a budget to buy further items of medical care (eg hospital treatment) for its registered patients on the open market, using its own discretion as to how the money is spent. The NHS and Community Care Act (effective from 1993) has set up a provision for funding multi-partner practices wanting to take on this extra management role in order to influence the quality of specialized services provided for their patients and to attempt to make a 'profit' which would benefit in-practice services

fungus a form of microscopic vegetable life which can be parasitic on man and cause disease

furuncle (boil) area of inflammation around a hair follicle where pus gathers and stretches the skin, which may eventually burst or need to be surgically opened

gall-bladder *see* **bladder**

gangrene death of the tissue in a part of the body; caused by loss of blood supply, especially in old people, or infection of the damaged tissue in a severe wound; amputation is usually necessary as the affected area becomes toxic

gastrectomy operation performed to remove a gastric ulcer or tumour in the stomach, or to remove the entire stomach in cases of advanced cancer. **gastroscopy** visual inspection of the interior of the stomach using a gastroscope (specialized endoscope, page 41)

gastroenteritis inflammation of the stomach and intestines causing diarrhoea and vomiting

gastroenterology the medical specialism concerned with conditions of the stomach and intestines

General Consultants' and Specialists' Committee (GCSC) a British Medical Association body which advises and negotiates with the Government on behalf of consultants and other specialist doctors

general dental practitioner (GDP) dentist who provides care to people in the community; GDPs are contracted to the FHSA in the same way as GMPs (below)

general manager a professional manager appointed to rationalize the operations of an NHS organization; such appointments were first made in response to the 1983 Griffiths report which criticized a lack of planning in the health services

General Medical Council (GMC) body set up as a 'watchdog' to ensure that professional standards are maintained by doctors; keeps a list of all registered (legally qualified) doctors, provides guidelines on expected standards of care, presides over cases of alleged misconduct, oversees educational standards and vets overseas doctors wishing to practice in the UK

General Medical Services Committee (GMSC) a British Medical Association body which advises and negotiates with the Government on behalf of GPs and other members of local medical committees (LMCs)

general (medical) practitioner (GP or GMP) a doctor who is specially qualified to provide health care to people in the community who present with a wide variety of medical (and psychological) problems; a working GP is essentially self-employed but is contracted (often in association with 'partners' – *see* page 66) to his/her local FHSA to provide a specified range of services to patients in a given area (GPs are said to have 'independent contractor status'); alternatively a person qualified to be a GP may work as a **restricted principal** (page 74), an assistant or a **locum** (page 56)

General Practice Contract (1990) contract which binds GPs to provide certain services; 1990 revisions redefine the GP's role, placing greater emphasis on health promotion and disease prevention – includes provision for regular check-ups for registered patients, especially the elderly, target levels of inoculation, development of health promotion clinics and child surveillance programmes, and minor surgery performed by the GP (*see* **item-of-service fees**)

generic of a drug, referring to its 'general' or 'real' name that describes its contents, as opposed to a brand name of a manufacturer (many drugs are known by the name of the most commonly used brand, eg Disprin). **generic prescribing** issuing of a drug order to a patient which specifies (to the pharmacist) a type of drug rather than the best-known brand; becoming more common because it can save money where different brands vary in cost

genes the units, each a coiled segment of the chemical deoxyribonucleic acid (DNA), that individually determine all inherited characteristics – both physical and mental; carried by chromosomes in the nucleus of every cell in the body. **genetics** the study of gene behaviour, particularly in relation to inherited diseases

geriatrics the medical specialism concerned with the diseases of old age, and with the general health and care of the elderly

German measles *see* **rubella**

giardiasis acute illness resulting from parasites in the gut which cause watery diarrhoea, flatulence and distension; can persist for six weeks or more; common in children

gigantism excessive growth, especially in height, caused by over-secretion of the pituitary growth hormone so that a tumour forms

gland an organ that secretes a substance, eg hormone, useful to the body; *see* **endocrine system, hormones** and page 15. **lymph gland** tissue adapted to filter lymph; *see* **lymph**

glandular fever *see* **infectious mononucleosis**

glans penis the bulbous tip of the penis

glucose tolerance test (GTT) test to detect diabetes; after a period of fasting the patient is given a quantity of glucose; the doctor can then measure the extent to which the body is able to stabilize its blood sugar level by naturally excreting insulin. Diabetics require administration of insulin or a careful diet to reduce absorption of sugars into the blood; *see also* **diabetes**

glue ear the commonest form of middle ear infection in children, causing deafness due to an accumulation of a glue-like substance

goitre an enlargement of the thyroid gland which results in a swollen neck; the gland's normal rate of hormone production may be disturbed by a deficiency of iodine

gonads the sex glands, situated in men in the testes and in women in the ovaries, which secrete the hormones testosterone and oestrogen/progesterone respectively

gonorrhoea complement fixation test (GCFT) blood test for the parasite which causes the sexually transmitted disease 'gonorrhoea'

gout a disease which causes painful swelling in the cartilages of the joints and ears due to an increase of uric acid in the blood;

results from an inability to deal with substances found in, for example, caffein and beer; may be hereditory or acquired due to over-indulgence

Graafian follicle *see* **ova**

grey matter collections of nerve cells in the brain and spinal cord

growth hormone (GH) hormone secreted by the pituitary gland at the base of the skull, which accelerates physical development during childhood

gullet *see* **oesophagus**

Guthrie's test estimation of the level of a protein (phenylalanine) in the blood by a urine test or pin prick in the heel within the first week of life, to detect a rare but severe form of mental deficiency (which can be reversed by diet if detected early enough)

gynaecology the medical specialism that is concerned with women's health and the conditions peculiar to women

haematocrit *see* **packed cell volume**

haemoglobin (Hb) a pigment in red blood cells (erythrocytes), which gives them their colour and whose function is to attract oxygen for the red blood cells to transport around the body. **haemoglobin estimation** test for lowered/excessive oxygen carrying capacity, which may indicate disease, eg anaemia/polycythaemia (excess of red blood cells) respectively

haemophilia a hereditory disease, affecting males only, which causes even minor wounds to bleed profusely owing to deficient blood clotting (coagulating) mechanism

Haemophilus influenza **type B (Hib)** a bacteria which causes serious infections in children, mostly commonly meningitis; *see* page 59

haemorrhage an incidence of excessive bleeding, usually occurring during or after an injury or operation

haemorrhoids (piles) formation of varicose veins in or around the anus, which may cause bleeding, pain or itching; may occur due to strain caused by constipation or during pregnancy

hallux valgus (HV) common outward deflection of the big toe, often causing a bunion to form

hammer toe common deformity of the second toe, in which the joints bend in different directions, and which is often aggravated by misfitting shoes

hay fever see **allergic rhinitis**

Heaf test test for susceptibility to TB; tiny amount of tuberculin bacterium is injected into the skin at multiple sites, and will cause redness if test is positive

health promotion an increasingly important responsibility of health workers, which involves educating the public and encouraging them to adopt a healthy lifestyle – eg with regard to diet, smoking and excercise. Regular health promotion clinics in general practices have been encouraged by the introduction of a special service payment to GPs

health visitor (HV) a specialist nurse employed by the District Health Authority, to visit vunerable groups in their homes, especially young mothers and their children, in order to advise them (on a medical and psychosocial basis) and assess how they are coping; may be 'attached' to a general practice (page 26)

hepatitis inflammation of the liver: (a) from a viral infection; (b) **infective hepatitis** (acute type A) from infected blood absorbed through mucous membranes of mouth, lips, etc; (c) **serum hepatitis** (acute type B) from contact with infected blood during transfusion or from needle-sharing among drug addicts

hereditory a characteristic or disease which is passed through a gene from parent to child; *cf* **acquired** and **congenital**

hermaphrodite rare abnormality in which the external sex organs are of one gender and hormones are produced that belong to the other (transexuals, who 'feel' like members of the other sex, are pseudo-hermaphrodites)

hernia protrusion of an organ or part of an organ through the wall of a body cavity (hollow); applies especially to the abdominal cavity, where a hernia or 'rupture' may in certain cases appear as a swelling in the groin. **hiatus hernia** protrusion of the stomach through the diaphragm. **hernioplasty** an operation to repair a hernia

herpes simplex (cold sore) a viral skin infection, which causes blistering on the face, often in conjunction with a common cold

herpes zoster (shingles) infection of nerve endings which causes blistering under the skin and stinging pain

hiatus hernia *see* **hernia**

histology microscpic study of the structures of tissues (collections of cells) in the body

HIV (human immunodeficiency virus) the virus that leads to AIDS; may lie dormant in the body, without any symptoms of disease, for an estimated 5–10 years

holistic an alternative philosphy of medicine which advocates the treatment of the whole person, including mental and social factors, rather than just the presenting disease

homoeopathy treatment of disease by minute doses of drugs that in a healthy person would produce symptoms of the disease

hormones substances secreted by glands situated in various parts of the body, which stimulate essential activities such as growth, metabolism (converting foods for energy and use in the body), and sexual functions. The functioning of glands operates within the **endocrine system**: *see* page 15. **hormone replacement therapy (HRT)** a treatment for women suffering from menopausal symptoms; involves administering regular doses of the female hormones with the effect of rejuvinating the patient

humerus the bone in the upper arm

hyperglycaemia excessive sugar in the blood; *see* **diabetes mellitus**

hypermetropia longsightedness, caused by faulty accommodation of the eye so that light is focused beyond instead of on the retina

hypertension sustained high blood pressure (force with which blood is pumped into the arteries from the heart) associated with excessive stress or obesity

hyperthyroidism *see* **thyroid gland**

hypertrophy excessive tissue growth

hypochondria a state of imagining one suffers from a physical illness

hypodermic relating to the area immediately beneath the skin. **hypodermic syringe** syringe used to inject drugs beneath the skin

hypothyroidism *see* **thyroid gland**

hysterectomy surgical removal of the uterus (womb), necessary in cases of cancerous or other tumours or occasionally excessive menstruation

hysteria neurotic state of uncontrollable emotion

immunization administration of modified disease-causing bacteria, orally or by injection, which stimulate production of antibodies that give immunity (prevent the disease from striking in the future); GPs routinely conduct immunization programmes for infectious diseases, which are offered to patients on their lists

impotence *see* **sterility**

incontinence lack of control over when urine or faeces are voided

incubation period the initial stage of a disease during which no symptoms present, ie the patient is effectively well; some diseases are characterized by an incubation period of a particular length

independent contractor status *see* **general practitioner**

independent medical adviser (IMA) person appointed by a Family Health Services Authority to advise on amounts to be set aside for GP prescribing; *see* **indicative prescribing**

indicative prescribing scheme for reducing the cost to the NHS of prescriptions made at a standard charge to patients; the Family Health Services Authority (page 43) specifies an annual practice budget (individualized for each practice based on factors such as list size), and the practice's prescribing habits are investigated if it overspends

induction of labour use of medical or surgical procedures to start the labour process in a woman at full term of pregancy

infectious disease a disease, caused by a micro-organism (bacterium, virus, fungus or protozoon) which is communicable, ie it may be passed from person to person

infectious mononucleosis (glandular fever) an infectious disease caused by a virus and which results in sore throat, high temperature and swelling of lymph glands; *see* page 14

inflammation swelling, tenderness and heating up of a part of the body as a reaction to injury or disease

influenza viral infection of the nose, throat and upper respiratory tract

insulin a substance (hormone) secreted from the pancreas, which enables the conversion of carbohydrates from food into energy; may be artifically administered to diabetics, who have insufficient natural secretions

intensive care medical treatment, with constant monitoring, of a dangerously ill patient; ward or department of hospital set aside for this

intravenous (IV) literally 'into a vein'; applied to an injection or an infusion (a 'drip') of fluids from a vessel, eg of nutrients.

intravenous cholangiogram X-ray, involving injection of a contrast medium to show up any obstructions (growths or stones) in the common bile duct

intravenous pylogram (IVP) X-ray, involving injection of a contrast medium to show functioning of kidneys and detect malfunction/disease

in-vitro fertilization artificial method of conception, whereby one or more ova are removed from the ovaries of the would-be mother and fertilized in a laboratory, then implanted in the womb

involuntary muscles muscles that operate bodily functions outside the conscious control of the individual; ie those in the walls of the circulatory, digestive, excretory and reproductive organs, and the heart muscle

iris the part of the eye that gives it its colour; contraction of its muscle controls the amount of light entering the eye

irritable bowel mild inflammatory disorder of the large intestine (colon) causing discomfort, for which there is no known cause; may be psychological

isotope radio-active substance used to trace the movement of chemical substances in the body (to make a diagnosis), or in research or treatment

item-of-service fees general practice income from fees for temporary resident care, emergency treatment, minor surgery, maternity medical services (MMS), contraception and night visits; plus immunizations (for over six-year-olds) and health promotion clinics for which fees are paid according to a lower or higher target percentage of the practice population that has been reached

jaundice yellow colouration of the skin and mucous membranes due to an excess of a bile pigment called bilirubin in the blood

Joffroy's sign test for diagnosing hyperthyroidism, the excessive excretion of the hormone from the thyroid gland

joints points at which two or more bones join together: **ball and socket joints** are found in the hip and shoulder and allow the bones to be rotated in a circular motion; **pivot joints** are found at the top of the spine and allow movement around one axis (vertical line); **hinge joints** are found in the knee and elbow; **gliding joints** in the hands and feet; **saddle joints** in the wrist and ankle

Kernig's sign test for meningitis or brain haemorrhage: inability to straighten leg, when patient is supine with thigh flexed, indicates disease

kidneys two organs situated either side of the spine, each about five inches long and bean-shaped, wherein blood is processed to remove the substances that make up urine; the urine is constantly carried from the kidneys along tubes called ureters to the urinary bladder. **kidney (renal) disease/failure** loss of kidney function, resulting in accumulation of urine in the bloodstream which untreated will eventually cause death. **renal dialysis** use of a machine to enact the kidneys' function, extracting waste from the blood at regular intervals in patients suffering from renal (kidney) disease. **kidney stones** (renal calculus) accumulations of calcium in the hollow of the kidney which may cause sharp pains, obstruct the ureter or pass into the bladder

Kilocalorie (Calorie) unit of energy used to measure the amount of nutrient transferrable into energy (or fat if it is not 'burned') from foods; much food packaging now displays this information, particularly for those who wish to lose weight by means of a 'calorie controlled diet'. **kilojoule** unit more commonly used by food scientists now; 1 kilocalorie = 4.2 kilojoules

knee jerk (KJ) test of patient's reflexes by striking the loose hanging leg just below the kneecap (patella) with a 'patella hammer'; normally it will jerk forward, and failure to do so may indicate disease of the central nervous system

Koplik's spots blue-white spots in the mouth, which appear on the third day after contracting measles

Kveim test injection of Kviem antigen into skin to diagnose sarcoidosis (page 75)

labyrinth test a diagnostic test which notes abnormal response to water in the ears as an indicator of nervous disease

laparoscopy internal examination of the abdomen/pelvic area using a fine flexible lighted tube passed into the body (an endoscope, or specifically a **laparoscope**) to investigate lower abdominal pain. **laparotomy** surgery through the abdominal wall; usually an exploratory procedure

laryngitis inflammation of the voice-box (larynx) and vocal cords resulting in dryness and hoarseness, tickling cough and raised temperature; may occur after exposure to an irritant, to the cold, or due to overuse of voice. **laryngoscopy** visual examination of the vocal cords, epiglottis and larynx, to detect paralysis of vocal cords, growths or infection, using a fine, flexible tube called a **laryngoscope**

larynx the voice-box

laser surgery transmission of energy as heat which can change the structure of tissue; used to treat skin cancer and detached retina

latex fixation test blood test for diagnosing rheumatoid arthritis

laxative drug that stimulates the movement of the bowels

lesion a diseased section of tissue (changed in its structure)

leukaemia a type of cancer (malignant growth); permanent excess of white blood cells which causes enlargement of the spleen and lymph glands all over the body, and changes in the bone marrow; some types (depending on the type of blood cells affected) are fatal if not treated; acute forms treated with **chemotherapy** (page 32)

ligaments stong fibrous bands of elastic tissue which connect bones or cartilages and support and strengthen joints

linctus a syrupy medicine such as a soothing cough mixture

liver the largest organ in the body, located in the upper right-hand side of the abdomen; secretes bile, an aid to digestion, and metabolizes (converts) sugars, fats and proteins for use in the body; also breaks down any poisons taken into the body, such as alcohol. **liver function tests (LFTs)** series of tests designed to detect liver disease or jaundice

locum doctor employed by a GP to assist him/her on an occasional or temporary basis, eg to 'cover' for his/her absence due to holiday or illness

lower respiratory tract consists of the windpipe, bronchi (tubes to the lungs), lungs and pleura (the membrane covering the lungs); cf **upper respiratory tract** and see also page 8

lumbago pain and/or muscular spasm in the 'small' of the back

lumbar puncture (LP) (spinal tap) extraction of cerebrospinal fluid (CSF) from between the 2nd and 3rd lumbar vertebrae for examination in order to detect certain diseases of the nervous system, eg meningitis. **cisternal puncture** alternative test, if lumbar puncture not possible; fluid taken from an opening in the base of the skull

lungs two cone-shaped organs of the respiratory system, located either side of the heart and consisting of air-sacs called alveoli which are surrounded by capillaries through which oxygen and carbon dioxide pass in and out of the body

lung scan test using radio-isotopes to diagnose tumours; *see* **isotope**

lymph fluid similar to plasma, but containing only one type of cell called a **lymphocyte** – a constituent of white blood cells which produces antibodies to limit the impact of infections, and filters and destroys bacteria; manufactured in **lymphoid tissue**, which is contained in **lymph glands** – *see* page 14 for primary locations. **lymphatic system** consists of lymph, lymph glands and lymph vessels which transport lymphocytes, as well as fluid, proteins and emulsified fat in the lymph, into the circulation. **thoracic duct** and **right lymphatic duct** the primary collection sites for lymph. **lymphangiography** X-ray of lymph vessels; enlargement may indicate pelvic cancer or Hodgkin's disease

macules areas of skin which have turned to a purple-brown colour, sometimes due to disease

malabsorption tests include sugar tolerance test, examination of faeces or tissue from bones or intestines; to diagnose impaired ability to absorb particular nutrients from the digestive tract

malaise condition of feeling unwell

malignant of a growth/tumour, harmful tissue which invades and destroys healthy tissue;. cancerous

mallet finger deformity which restricts finger movement

mammary glands (breasts) secondary sexual organs whose production of milk at the end of pregnancy is stimulated by a hormone released from the pituitary gland; *see* page 15

mammography X-ray of soft tissue in the breast to detect early malignancy

Mantoux test test for susceptibility to TB; tiny amount of tuberculin bacterium is injected into the skin and will cause redness if test is positive

mastectomy removal of the breast(s), usually when it is cancerous; may be 'simple' (removal of breast tissue and skin only) or 'radical' (removal of breast and underlying muscle and lymphoid tissue) if the cancer has spread to the glands

mastication chewing, the first stage of digestion

mean corpuscular volume (MCV), mean corpuscular haemoglobin (MCH), mean corpuscular haemoglobin concentration (MCHC) laboratory tests on red blood cells for diagnosing diseases characterized by red cell/haemoglobin content of blood above or below the normal ranges

measles *see* **morbilli**

Medical Audit Advisory Group (MAAG) set up by each Family Health Services Authority to monitor the quality of clinical service and obtain data for clinical audit (page 26)

Medical Defence Union (MDU) body which offers insurance to doctors, eg for legal proceedings for medical negligence/ accidents or failure of a partnership etc; almost all GPs subscribe to a medical defence body, usually either the MDU or the **Medical Protection Society (MPS)**

Medical Protection Society *see* **Medical Defence Union**

Medical Reports Act (1988) legislation giving patients right of access to medical reports prepared by a doctor

meiosis division of cells in the reproductive organs, ie in the testes and ovaries, with new cells containing half the number of chromosomes as their parent cell (when fertilized the chromosomes from the male and female cells form a new 'individual'); *see also* **chromosomes**

melanin dark pigment produced in skin, hair and the iris in the eye, particularly as a protective response to sunlight, ie tanning. **melanoma** tumour arising from melanin-producing cells; may be 'simple', ie a mole, or malignant, ie cancerous

membrane a thin lining (to organs and cells)

meningitis inflammation of the membranes surrounding the brain and spinal cord, called the **meninges**, due to a bacterial or viral infection and causing fever

menopause cessation of menstruation at the end of a woman's possible reproductive years, usually at age 45–50 years

menstruation monthly discharge of blood from the womb of a sexually mature woman (who is not pregnant), controlled by hormones released from the pituitary gland and ovaries

Mental Health Commission (MHC) established under the Mental Health Act 1983, and responsible for protecting the rights of patients detained under this Act

metabolism the continual series of chemical changes in the body, by which life is maintained, ie breakdown of food for conversion into energy, production of substances to stimulate growth, etc. **metabolic rate** the speed at which an individual 'uses up' energy intake (ie 'burns' calories)

metacarpals the bones in the hands

metatarsals the bones in the feet

microbiology the study of tiny living organisms called **microorganisms** (only visible through a microscope), eg bacteria and viruses that cause disease

micturition the act of passing urine

midstream specimen of urine *see* **catheter specimen of urine**

midwife specialist nurse qualified to give care during pregnancy, to assist in the process of childbirth and to care for the
mother and her new baby; may be based in the community and
attached to a general practice, or may be hospital-based

migraine severe headache often accompanied by vomiting and
preceeded by temporary disturbance of vision or other sensa-
tions; recurrent in sufferers

MIMS *see* **Monthly Index of Medical Specialties**

minimal access/minimally invasive of surgical procedures
involving a smaller incision into the body surface than tradi-
tional surgery; in particular the 'key-hole' method wherein the
scalpel enters the body attached to a long tube and is guided to
the diseased organ by means of a tiny camera; reduces time
patient needs to stay hospital

minor surgery surgery that may be undertaken by a GP using
equipment kept in-practice; currently encouraged (with incen-
tive payments) by the Department of Health to avoid the
unnecessary cost of referral to a hospital-based surgeon

mitosis cell reproduction; one cell divides into two identical
cells to achieve growth and repair of the tissue; *cf* **meiosis**

Moebius' sign test for diagnosing hyperthyroidism, the excessive excretion of the hormone from the thyroid gland

Monospot blood test to diagnose glandular fever

Monthly Index of Medical Specialties (MIMS) reference
manual, sent free to all GPs, that contains the names of all
proprietary drugs and their costs

morbidity state of being diseased, especially in relation to
statistics of disease in a population

morbilli (measles) infectious disease common in childhood and caused by a virus; symptoms are fever, catarrh, rash and Koplik's spots – see page 55

mortality death, especially in relation to population statistics, eg of causes/age

motor neurone disease degerative disease of the motor nerve in the spinal cord, resulting in gradual muscle wasting, usually in middle age

multigravida woman who has given birth more than once

multipara woman in her second or subsequent pregnancy; *cf* **primipara**

multiple sclerosis (MS) degenerative disease in which the muscle fibres in the brain and spinal cord are damaged by a virus and gradually destroyed; symptoms include impaired vision, weakness of limbs (patient may eventually become wheel-chair bound) and sometimes difficulty in urinating

mumps *see* **epidemic parotitis**

muscular dystrophy term applied to hereditory diseases characterized by gradual muscle wasting (atrophy) which results in disability or deformity; may occur in various groups of muscles

myelogram X-ray view of spinal canal by means of radio-opaque dye to detect tumours; *see also* **radiculography**

myopia short-sightedness, ie loss of clarity when looking into the distance; light rays come to a focus in front of, instead of on, the retina; correctable with spectacles

nasal swab sample of mucus taken from the nostrils to indentify carriers of the *Staphlococcus* bacterium which causes common infections

National Association of Health Authorities and Trusts (NAHAT) set up in 1990, primarily to express the collective views of Family Health Services Authorities (page 43) and NHS Trusts (page 83) on national issues

neck rigidity test that indicates meningeal irritation if neck flexion is limited

necrosis tissue death

neonate a baby up to four weeks old

neoplasm (literally 'new formation') a tumour or cyst

nephrectomy surgical removal of a diseased kidney

nerve-grafting procedure undertaken to fill a gap between nerve ends, using segments of a nerve from another part of the body, as in a skin graft

nervous system the structures which control all the body's functions; the **central nervous system** consists of the brain, spinal cord and **neurons** that connect the brain with every cell in the body to co-ordinate conscious movement via peripheral nerves; the **autonomic nervous system** comprises nerves that control unconscious acts, ie parasympathetic and sympathetic nerves – *see* page 16

neuralgia sharp stabbing pain along the course of a nerve, usually due to inflammation

neurology branch of medicine concerned with the nervous system and its diseases

neuron a nerve cell with accompanying **axon** (long fibre) which conveys impulses away from the cell and **dendrites** which convey impulses to it, and nerve endings (page 16). **motor nerves/ neurons** send messages from the brain to the muscles and **sensory nerves/neurons** send messages to the brain

NHS and Community Care Act (1991) programme of reforms instituted in response to the Government White Papers (research publications) *Caring for People* and *Working for*

Patients; mainly concerned with improving quality and efficiency in the local provision of health care services – *see* **audit, fundholding** and **indicative prescribing**

nucleus the control centre of every cell, which contains its genetic material

nuclear magnetic resonance imaging (NMRI) diagnostic technique employing radio frequency radiation in the presence of a magnetic field to produce anatomical sections of the body

nurse practitioner nurse who works in the community, attached to a general practice, but who is independent from the GP and is authorized to prescribe for certain conditions, *cf* **practice nurse**

obesity state of being overweight (storing excess fat) to the extent of endangering health

obstetrics branch of medicine concerned with pregancy, childbirth and associated care of the mother and new baby; including midwifery

oedema abnormal infiltration of fluid into tissue

oesophagus canal extending from the throat to the stomach, through which food passes and begins to be digested due to the contraction and relaxation of oesophageal muscles. **oesophagoscopy** endoscopic (through a lighted tube) investigation of the inner lining of the oesophagus, to check for tumours; may also be used to remove foreign bodies

oestrogen collective term for three female sex hormones secreted by the ovaries – oestriol, oestrone and oestradiol – which cause the body to reach and maintain sexual maturity, and prepare it for childbirth. **oestriol examination** examination of oestrogen in the urine during pregnancy, to check that fetus and placenta are functioning normally

oliguria diminished secretion of urine

ophthalmic pertaining to the eye. **ophthalmoscope** instrument fitted with a light and a lens for examining the interior of the eye to detect disease. **ophthalmologist** doctor specializing in diseases of the eyes

opportunistic screening disease prevention measure undertaken as an alternative to the three-yearly check-ups now recommended for those who would not otherwise see a doctor: patients who present with a specific problem are given a generalized check-up during which the doctor looks for indicators of future problems

optic nerve nerve entering the back of the eye, which transmits visual stimuli from the retina to the brain

optician person qualified to correct refractive problems, ie prescribe spectacles for those with short/long sight

oral cytology 'smear' sample taken from lesions (damaged tissue) in the mouth to check for malignancy

orthodontics branch of dentistry dealing with correction of irregularities of the teeth, eg fitting of braces

orthopaedics branch of surgery specializing in problems of movement/mobility

osteopathy 1. disease of the bones (generic) 2. bone manipulation to treat pain caused by skeleton being, allegedly, out of line; practised by non-doctors as an alternative to conventional treatment

osteoporosis condition where the bones become porous (lose their water-tight character); resultant loss of calcium causes them to become brittle, ie easily broken

otalgia earache

ovum (pl. **ova**) female reproductive cell ('egg'); released once a month from a **Graffian follicle** (in which each individual ovum is contained) in one of the ovaries of a sexually mature woman;

it travels along the **Fallopian tube** to the uterus (womb) where it may be ferilized or released from the body in mentruation. **ovaries** two organs, situated either side of the womb, in which the ova are produced; *see* Figure 9. **ovulation** process of expulsion of an ovum from the ovary

pacemaker 1. region in the heart that initiates its muscle contractions and controls their rate 2. artificial device implanted to perform this action

packed cell volume (PCV) (haematocrit) computerized laboratory test of the proportion in the blood of packed red cells; abnormally high or low levels may indicate disease

PACT data *see* **Prescribing Analyses and Costs**

paediatrics specialism concerned with children and childhood disease. **paediatrician** doctor qualified in paediatrics

Paget's disease (osteitis deformans) skeletal collapse and deformity caused by defective new bone formation; affects mainly old men

palatal reflex test wherein the soft palate at the back of the roof of the mouth is touched and normally activates reflex rising, except if the patient has an hysterical condition

palliative care nursing with the object of alleviating pain or discomfort and improving quality of life; especially refers to cases of incurable terminal illness, eg in a hospice

palpitations strong rapid beating of the heart of which patient is conscious

pancreas organ situated below and behind the stomach (*see* page 10) containing enzymes that assist in digestion by secreting insulin into the bloodstream – a substance necessary for converting sugars for use in the body (lack of insulin can cause diabetes mellitus)

papules pimples, 'spots'

paracentesis (aspiration) withdrawal of a sample of fluid from a part of the body (by means of suction or siphon) to test for disease. **ascitic fluid** paracentesis of fluid in the abdomen to test for heart, liver or kidney failure

paraplegia paralysis of the lower trunk, including the bladder and rectum, and the legs

Parkinson's disease degenerative nervous disease, affecting mainly old people, which gives rise to symptoms of muscular rigidity and tremor in the face and limbs, and a shuffling gait

partnership arrangement wherein two or more fully qualified GPs share premises, workload and profits; partners make joint decisions regarding practice policy, and although each doctor usually has his/her own list of patients (often by the latter's choice), partners will see each other's patients

patella the kneecap

patella hammer *see* **knee jerk**

Patient's Charter Government statement (1992) of the rights of NHS patients as 'consumers' of health care services, and of standards of behaviour towards patients that health service providers should adhere to; restates recognized rights such as access to medical care regardless of ability to pay, and introduces new 'rights' which reflect a policy of freedom to make informed choices. The main items on the agenda are: provision of detailed information to patients and their families; guaranteed maximum waiting times; the right to regular health checks, especially for children and the elderly; the right to have a complaint heard or to change doctors; and respect for individual needs

pathology study of the causes and characteristics of disease

Paul Bunnel test blood test to diagnose glandular fever

peak flow gauge instrument used to detect rate of expiration in an asthmatic, ie the 'peak expiratory flow rate' (PEFR) – measurement of this shows the degree of resistance to airflow from the lungs

pediculosis capitalis head lice. **pediculosis corporis** lice on the body. **pediculosis pubis** lice in the pubic hair

pelvis basin-shaped lower part of the abdominal cavity created by the pelvic girdle of bones which surround the bladder, rectum and (in women) the reproductive organs; *see* page 7

pemphigus diseases which cause a blistery eruption on the skin and mucous membranes

peptic ulcer an ulcer in the stomach or duodenum (the first portion of the small intestine)

peripheral nerves *see* **nervous system**

peristalsis force which brings about a pattern of contraction and relaxation in the intestines in order to move food along as it is digested

pernicious anaemia *see* **anaemia**

pertussis (whooping cough) infectious childhood disease which causes long exhausting episodes of coughing and choking, sometimes leading to more serious repercussions

pessary 1. medication for insertion into the vagina to treat an infection or as a contraceptive 2. an instrument inserted into the vagina to correct a displaced womb

petechiae small red spots on the skin, formed by effusion (escape) of blood

phalanges bones of the fingers and toes

pharmacology the study of drugs and their effects on the body.
pharmacy the preparation and dispensing of medicinal drugs.
pharmacist person qualified to practise pharmacy

pharynx the throat – cavity lined with a slippery mucous membrane, which functions in respiration (part of the upper respiatory tract) and digestion (swallowing)

phobia an irrational fear; eg **agoraphobia** fear of open spaces; **claustrophobia** fear of confined spaces; **arachnophobia** fear of spiders

phonocardiogram recording of heart sounds on a graph in order to interpret heart murmurs

physiology the study of the body's functions

physiotherapy treatment of injury, disease or deformity by physical methods, such as manipulation, massage or prescribed exercise; usually by referral from the patient's doctor to a qualified physiotherapist

pituitary gland endocrine gland (*see* page 15) at the base of the skull, whose anterior and posterior lobes secrete various hormones into the bloodstream which stimulate growth and play a part in kidney regulation, development of the sex glands, childbirth and production of milk for breast-feeding; malfunction of either lobe can be assessed by laboratory tests

placenta (the 'afterbirth') organ which forms against the inner wall of the womb in the third month of pregnancy; supplies the fetus with nourishment from the mother via the umbilical cord; expelled from the body about an hour after the birth

plantar reflex test for nervous disease wherein the sole of the foot is stimulated; normal response is automatic curling of the toes, but upturn of big toe only (**Babinski's sign**) indicates a disorder of the central nervous system

plasma the fluid base of blood, mostly water but also containing proteins, mineral salts, antibodies and secretions from the endocrine glands

platelets (thrombocytes) the cells in blood that cause it to clot at the site of an injury to prevent excessive bleeding. **platelet count** laboratory test; if proportion of platelets in the blood is outside the normal range, disease may be indicated

pleura a lubricating lining, consisting of two layers around the inside of the lungs; also line the ribs. **pleurisy** inflammation of the pleura and discharge of fluid into the cavity between pleural layers (in lungs). **pleural fluid** can be drawn off for examination to diagnose malignancy, chest injury, TB or heart failure. **pneumonia** inflammation of lung tissue – causing air sacs to fill with pus – due to bacterial or viral infection, usually as a result of prolonged exposure to cold

polio virus which causes poliomyelitis, wherein nerves in the brain stem and spinal cord are attacked, and the patient becomes paralysed

polyuria the passing of excessive amounts of urine

posterior the surface area of the back of the body

postgraduate education allowance (PGEA) scheme for reimbursing GPs for their costs in undertaking recognized educational pursuits; a means of encouraging GPs to engage in continuing medical education (CME), particularly from the point of view of keeping up-to-date with new developments in medical research and practice

post-mortem (PM) an examination of the body after death, in order to determine the cause in suspicious or unusual circumstances

postnatal with reference to the first few weeks following childbirth

practice nurse nurse employed by a GP partnership to work in the practice, undertaking such tasks as first aid, immunizations and, especially since the 1990 General Practice Contract, conducting health promotion and chronic disease clinics, cervical smears and patient check-ups

premature baby a baby born before the 40th week of pregnancy, but mature enough to survive

Prescribing Analyses and Costs (PACT) computerized system used to calculate each GP's prescribing costs by category, type of drug and use; based on quarterly GP reports

primary care 'first contact' care of patients presenting with symptoms, usually to their GP or other health care worker in the community; *cf* **secondary care**

primigravida woman who has given birth for the first time; *cf* **multigravida**

primipara woman in her first pregnancy; *cf* **multipara**

proctocscopy visual examination of the rectum through a lighted tube (protoscope) for detection of haemorrhoids or growths, or tissue collection for biopsy

prodromal signs and symptoms which precede the full onset of a disease, eg a transitory rash

progesterone female sex hormone which prepares the uterus monthly for pregancy; when ovulation occurs (time of the month when an ovum is released from an ovary for possible fertilization) the pituitary gland also stimulates formation of a yellow mass called **corpus luteum**, which secretes progesterone

prognosis forecast of the probable course of a disease

prolapse collapse/falling of an organ out of its correct position. **prolapsed intervertebral disc (PID)** (slipped disc) layer of cartilage which has prolapsed ('slipped out') from between the vertebrae, usually in the lumbar region of the spine in the small of the back, which may cause pressure against a nerve and result in **lumbago** or **sciatica**. **uterine prolapse** fall of the uterus into the vagina. **rectocele** prolapse of the rectum so that it descends outside the anus

prostate gland small conical gland at the base of the male bladder; releases a fluid that forms part of the semen

prothrombin ratio blood test – of plasma clotting time – to investigate for haemorrhagic disorders (internal bleeding) or liver disease

providers/provider units literally those who directly 'provide' medical care; term used since the 1990 NHS and Community Care Act (page 62) to refer to NHS secondary care providers (mainly hospitals) whose services are 'purchased' by District Health Authorities for patients in a catchment area, or directly by fundholding practices (page 44) for their registered patients; *see also* **Trusts**

pruritus itching

psoriasis hereditory chronic skin disease; affected sites – often knees and elbows – become roughened, red, scaley and itchy

psychiatry the study of mental illness, and its diagnosis and treatment; psychiatrists are medically qualified and permitted to prescribe drugs. **psychology** behaviourial study, in practice often dealing with mentally ill subjects; clinical psychologists are medically qualified, but do not prescribe drugs. **psycho-therapy** a type of social work specializing in mental illness

psychosis severe mental disease which affects all aspects of the personality

puerpurium the period of approximately six weeks following childbirth, until ovulation has occurred

pulmonary pertaining to the lungs. **pulmonary artery** the main artery leaving the heart, which carries de-oxygenated ('used') blood to the lungs. **pulmonary vein** returns oxygenated blood to the heart from the lungs; *see* Figure 5

pulse a rhythmic beat which can be detected in arteries near the body's surface, such as the radial artery in the wrist and the carotid artery in the neck; caused by the heart's 'pumping' action which sends an impulse through all the arteries

pupil the black centre of the eye, a hole into which light passes and makes contact with the lens behind; the pupils can contract (narrow) or become enlarged under the control of an involuntary muscle in order to restrict or increase the amount of light entering the eye. **pupil reflex tests** (a) light is flashed in the eyes to check pupil contraction (b) patient is asked to look alternately at distant and near objects for assessment of normal pupil contraction; abnormal responses may indicate disease of the central nervous system

purchaser organization which buys medical care for NHS patients under its jurisdiction; *see* **fundholding** and **provider**

purpura skin condition wherein blood escapes from surface capillaries into the skin, giving the appearance of patches of small red spots or purple 'bruises'

purulent pertaining to or ressembling pus, which is a yellowish substance that contains bacteria and forms at the site of infections

pustule pimple containing pus

pyelitis an infection causing inflammation of the pelvis (basin-shaped cavity); a common complication in pregancy

pyrexia fever (not specific to any disease)

pyuria pus in urine

quality adjusted life year (QALY) method of determining priorities by assessing cost-benefits (whether the benefits obtained from a treatment justify the cost); calculations are made of costs in relation to the number of years of life saved and the quality of life given

radiculography similar procedure to myelography, to investigate lumbo-sacral nerve roots in the spine

radiography (X-rays) painless method of investigating parts of the body not visible on the surface, by passing waves of electromagnetic energy into the affected part to obtain a 'picture'; usually performed to diagnose bone fractures or disease; sometimes 'contrast media' are used to look at organs or soft tissue. **radiology** the study of the diagnosis of disease from X-rays

radius the thinner of the two bones of the forearm

rapid plasma reagin (RPR) blood test to diagnose venereal disease

rectum the lower part of the large intestine inside which faeces are stored pending expulsion from the body

red blood corpuscles/cells (RBC) (erythrocytes) a type of blood cell which is formed in bone marrow; RBCs contain a protein called globin and iron, and part of the used RBC is recycled into bilirubin (a constituent of bile). **red blood cell count** laboratory test to check that the proportion of red cells in the blood is within the normal range; raised levels may indicate dyhydration whereas lowered levels may indicate haemorrhaging (internal bleeding)

Red Book commonly used name for the Department of Health's Statement of Fees and Allowances which sets out the basis on which GPs are paid and practices financed

reflex involuntary muscle reaction to a sensory stimulus, eg corneal reflex, a reaction of blinking when the cornea (outer covering of the eye) is touched

refraction the bending of light rays so that the image of an object is focused, in normal sight on the retina (the eye's inner nervous tissue). **refraction tests** the 'trying out' of various corrective lenses until a person has full vision

Regional Health Authority (RHA) NHS body (14 in England and Wales) directly accountable to the Secretary of State for Health, which is responsible for planning and allocation of resources (including building projects), implementing government reforms and overseeing District Health Authority (page 39) and Family Health Services Authority (page 43) activities, and regulating purchaser-provider transactions (*see* pages 72 and 71)

renal (failure, transplant etc) *see* **kidneys**

renal biopsy obtaining of renal tissue by puncture, rather than open operation, for examination

reproductive system in a woman consists of the ovaries, uterus, Fallopian tubes, vagina and vulva; and in a man, the testes, vas deferens, prostate gland, seminal vessels and penis (*see* individual entries)

respiratory system (RS) the organs and tissues concerned with breathing; these involve exchange of oxygen and carbon dioxide (and water vapour) between the body's cells and the outside environment by means of blood circulation and the lungs (*see* Figure 4). The organs used in breathing comprise the **upper respiratory tract** (the nose, throat and larynx) and the **lower respiratory tract** (the trachea, bronchi and lungs) (*see* individual entries)

restricted principle official term describing a GP who is fully qualified but whose contract limits his/her range of activities, eg might apply to a GP who works only in a family planning clinic

retina the light-sensitive inner coating of the eyeball, mainly consisting of nervous tissue and on which light rays normally converge

Rhesus factor (Rh) *see* **agglutinogen**

rheumatism term referring to diseases which cause pain and swelling in muscles and joints (eg *see* **arthritis, rheumatoid**);

in acute 'rheumatic fever' accompanied by a bacterial throat infection

rhinoscopy visual examination, using a lighted tube, of the interior of the nose, and removal of tissue samples for testing

ribs there are 12 pairs, attached to the vertebrae and, excepting four 'floating ribs', to the sternum

ringworm fungal infection of the skin, characterized by circular scaly patches

Rinne's test test for deafness originating from the middle ear; involves use of a tuning fork (page 83)

Romberg's sign test for detecting impaired co-ordination – which might indicate multiple sclerosis or a cerebral tumour – wherein the patient is asked to stand with feet together and eyes closed

Rose-Waaler test blood test to diagnose rheumatoid arthritis

rubella (German measles) acute, infectious disease caused by a virus and resulting in fever and rash; common in children and only serious when contracted during the early months of pregnancy, when the fetus may be deformed

sacrum triangular bone formed of five vertebrae fused together, situated above the coccyx at the base of the back

salivary glands glands that secrete saliva into the mouth to soften food and thus facilitate chewing and swallowing

sarcoidosis chronic, TB-like inflammation of unknown origin; may affect the lungs, liver, spleen, skin, eyes, etc; sometimes resolves without causing damage

scabies skin infestation with the parasitic itch mite, which causes severe itching and a rash

scan investigation (for tumours) of internal organs, eg of the brain, bones, breasts or lungs, by building up an image from movement across the tissue, often involving injection of an element called radio-isotope to facilitate tracing

scarlatina (scarlet fever) infectious disease, mainly affecting children, which is caused by a *Streptococcus* bacterium and results in sore throat, fever and a rash on the trunk

Schick test test for susceptibility to diphtheria; a tiny amount of diphtheria toxin is injected into the skin and will cause a reaction if test is positive

Schilling test test for malabsorption of vitamin B_{12}, which is an indicator for pernicious anaemia

sciatica pain in the sciatic nerve which runs through the backs of the legs

sclera the 'white' of the eye; its outer layer including the transparent cornea at the front

screening generic name for a system of identifying disease, eg by examination and scanning using a fluorescent screen

scrotum pouch which contains the testes and epididymides (*see* Figure 8)

secondary care patient care occurring at a centralized establishment (hospital) or at the hands of a specialist, often as a result of a GP referral, as opposed to the first contact ('primary') care provided by a generalist local doctor (GP) or nurse

seminal vesicles two small sacs at the back of the male bladder, which secrete a fluid that, in combination with spermatozoa, forms semen

sensation tests methods of detecting disease of the central nervous system, by testing response to touch, heat, cold and pain

septic infected by pus-producing organisms, eg occurs when a wound is not cleaned; *see also* **antiseptic**

septicaemia blood-poisoning, with bacteria living in the blood

sex hormones secretions (*see* **hormones**) from the male/female sex glands which prepare the body for reproduction by stimulating gender-specific functions, especially at puberty; the principal sex hormones are, in women, oestrogen and progesterone, and in men, testosterone

sickle-cell anaemia *see* **anaemia**

sigmoidoscopy visual examination, through a lighted tube, of the interior of the sigmoid colon, to detect ulcerative colitis or amoebic dysentery

simple melanoma a mole; *see also* **melanin**

shingles see **herpes zoster**

slipped disc *see* **prolapse**

small intestine coiled tube (part of alimentary canal, *see* Figure 6) into which semi-liquid food ('chyme') passes from the stomach and is further digested by chemical secretions from the liver, gall-bladder and pancreas; nutrients are then absorbed by capillaries and lymph vessels and waste products pass into the large intestine called the colon; consists of three sections called the **duodenum, jejunum** and **ileum**

Snellen's test test employing a card with letters of various sizes to determine the extent of the subject's field of vision (eg for spectacles prescription)

spasm a convulsive, involuntary muscle contraction

spermatazoon (pl. -zoa; 'sperm') a mature male reproductive cell, the active constituent of semen which fertilizes the female ovum

spina bifida a congenital (from birth) defect of the spine, in which two or more vertebrae are imperfectly joined ('bifid' means cleft, ie split open)

spinal cord nervous fibre (directly connected to the brain) which is enclosed within the upper vertebrae, running down to the 1st or 2nd lumbar vertebra

spleen organ at the base of the pancreas, behind the stomach, which is involved in maintaining the quality of circulating blood; can become enlarged/inflammed if blood is defective

spondylosis degeneration/gradual deformation of the discs (round flat cartilages) between the vertebrae, similar to osteo-arthritis – *see* **arthritis**

spontaneous abortion a 'miscarriage', ie involuntary expulsion and death of the fetus usually before the 28th week of pregnancy; may result from a fetal deformity or trauma to the mother

sprain injury to soft tissue surrounding a joint, causing swelling and pain

Stanford-Binet tests a series of age-related tests of mental development for children over two years old

Statement of Fees and Allowances *see* **Red Book**

sterility inability of male or female partner to produce offspring; distinct from 'impotence', the inability of a man to have sexual intercourse

sternum the 'breast' bone, situated just under the skin in the centre of the chest; protects the heart and is attached to the ribs

steroids group of drugs which contain sex hormones and vitamins and may be prescribed for skin conditions; also renowned for their strength-enhancing properties, hence their illegal use by bodybuilders

stethoscope instrument (frequently used by GPs) for listening to sounds made by the body, especially those of the heart and chest

stillbirth the birth of a dead child (in early pregnancy called 'miscarriage')

stomach pear-shaped organ in which food is partially digested and turned into 'chyme', a creamy-yellow acidic fluid

stools faeces or excrement, especially samples collected for investigation (for typhoid, paratyphoid, dysentery, parasites, or if contain blood for diagnosis of gastric/duodenal ulcers)

strabismus a squint, ie inco-ordination of the muscles in the two eyes, so that light rays converge on a different point for each eye

stress incontinence involuntary urination (especially at times of stress), in women often due to a weakness in the muscle of the urethra

stupor partial unconsciousness, eg after a blow to the head or intoxication with alcohol

STYCAR (Sheridan tests for young children and retards) tests to diagnose abnormally slow mental development or, alternatively, hearing/vision problems

subcutaneous tissue type of tissue which exists just under the dermis, comprising nerve endings which detect pressure and store fat; *see* Figure 16

supine lying flat on the (patient's) back, eg for physical examination or operative procedures

suppository drug or substance that is introduced into the body via the rectum, and which then melts at body temperature

suture a 'stitch' to seal a wound or operative incision

sweat test procedure to detect excessive salt in a baby's sweat (sample from forearm) which may indicate the presence of cystic fibrosis

syphilis a venereal disease (passed on by sexual intercourse), which initially results in inflammation of the genitals and then affects the skin, bones, muscles and brain

tachycardia abnormally rapid heart beat

tarsals the bones of the ankles; *see also* **metatarsals**

tendon fibrous cord by which a muscle is attached to bone. **tenogram** X-ray, using a contrast medium, of a tendon sheath, to ascertain whether it is functioning properly

terminal care care of people who are dying, ie those with incurable diseases; *see also* **palliative care**

testes two male reproductive organs in which spermatozoa and the male hormone testosterone are generated

testosterone the male sex hormone, formed in the testes and responsible for male characteristics such as muscle formation and aggressive personality traits

tetanus ('lockjaw') disease caused by a micro-organism found in animals and manure etc; may be caught if a cut comes into contact with such 'dirt', resulting in muscle spasms and fear of water; commonly inoculated against

thermography method of investigating tissue damage by measuring changes of temperature on the surface of the skin, eg to detect tumours in the breast or to assess the progress of wound healing

thermometer instrument used to measure body temperature in cases of suspected fever; mercury/alcohol expands along the glass tube when heated

thoracoscopy examination through a lighted tube (thoracoscope) of the pleura (linings of the lungs); for diagnosis of disease or division of adhesions (abnormal tissue union)

thorax the upper trunk. **thoracic cavity** a hollow in the thorax, bounded by thoracic vertebrae at the back, ribs at the sides and the sternum at the front; contains and protects the heart and lungs

throat swab a sample of fluid taken from the throat to diagnose infections

thrombocytes *see* **platelets**

thyroid glands comprise two lobes situated either side of the trachea (windpipe) (*see* Figure 11), which secrete into the bloodstream a chemical containing the hormone 'thyroxine' that controls the metabolism of foods which aid growth and repair; defective working of the gland can result in various mental and physical growth disorders. **thyroid function tests (TFTs)** laboratory blood tests which enable assessment of whether the gland is functioning properly. Excessive thyroid production is called **hyperthyroidism** or **thyrotoxicosis**, and is characterized by anxiety, sweating and weight loss, whereas reduced thyroid production is called **hypothyroidism** in adults (causing physical slowing down and mental dullness) or **cretinism** in children born with a deficiency (*see* page 37)

tibia (shin-bone) bone running down the front of the lower leg

tinea ringworm. **tinea capitis** headlice. **tinea pedis** athlete's foot, ie infection between the toes

tinnitus ringing in the ears

tissue a collection of cells which forms the substance of a part of the body; specialized types of tissue are adapted to particular functions; *see* pages 3–5

tomography X-ray technique for examining a single layer of tissue, which entails blurring on the film of the layers above and below the one to be studied. **computerized tomography (CT)** scanners can build up a three-dimensional image when the body is examined from many different angles; used for detecting lesions (diseased tissue) in the brain, thorax and abdomen

tongue depressor instrument commonly used to get the tongue out of the way in order to inspect the throat

tonsils two small masses of lymphoid tissue (fights infection) on either side of the throat. **tonsilitis** inflammation of the tonsils

toxaemia circulation of toxins in the blood. **toxaemia of pregnancy** raised blood pressure, swollen ankles, vomiting and headache caused by a protein (which may be detected in urine sample)

toxins poisons

trachea (windpipe) long tube made of cartilage and lined with mucous membrane which connects the larynx (voice-box) to the bronchi (tubes leading into the lungs); used as an air passage in breathing

transplant replacement of a diseased or damaged organ (eg heart, lung, kidney or liver) with a healthy one from a recently brain-dead donor, or from a healthy relative where appropriate

trauma bodily injury or emotional shock, eg from car crash

tremor involuntary shaking, especially during movement, which is a feature of some diseases, eg Parkinson's and multiple sclerosis, or can be induced by alcoholism or shock/fear

treponema pallidum haemoglutination test (TPHA) blood test to diagnose venereal disease

Trusts NHS hospitals which have opted to become self-governing – ie to take direct financial responsibility for providing a service to communities, rather than being managed by the District Health Authority; Trusts negotiate contracts (in competition with each other) with fundholding practices to treat patients at a specified cost; other hospitals or treatment centres are now known as **provider units** (page 71) and are becoming increasingly autonomous, many with the aim of eventually being given Trust status

tuberculosis (TB) (pulmonary TB) infectious disease of the lungs caused by a bacteria called 'tubercle bacillus'; children customarily given immunity to TB with a vaccine (BCG)

tumour swelling or growth of abnormal, useless tissue which spreads at the expense of the body; may be benign (of limited size) or malignant (liable to spread and damage organs)

tuning fork steel instrument which is struck against particular surfaces to produce different sounds; commonly used by GPs and ENT specialists to test for deafness

typhoid fever infectious disease caused by a strain of salmonella and usually spread by contamination of food or water with sewage (common in developing countries); symptoms include diarrhoea and a rash on the chest

ulcer destruction of a mucous membrane (lining an organ or hollow) or of the skin, producing a crater which swells and, if it penetrates a blood vessel, bleeds. **peptic ulcer (PU)** an ulcer in the stomach or duodenum (first section of the small intestine). **rodent ulcer (RU)** ulcer in the skin. **ulcerative colitis (UC)** an inflammed colon (large intestine) with ulcer(s), causing diarrhoea with blood and mucus

ulna the inner (larger) bone of the forearm

ultrasound investigation of the uterus (womb) to estimate fetal maturity, and to detect multiple births or any abnormality; waves transmit noises from inside the womb

ultrasound cardiograph (USC) *see* **echocardiograph**

umbilical cord tube attached to the fetus during pregnancy, which carries to it a blood supply from the mother and nourishment from the embryo (a mass attached to the uterine wall)

undescended testis a testis that has failed to descend into the scrotal sac (its normal location) shortly before birth

unresricted principle GP who, as is usual, may practice in an area without restriction on the scope of patients or conditions seen; *cf* **restricted principle**

upper respiratory tract the upper parts of the body through which gases pass en route to (and from) the lungs during breathing: the nose, pharynx (throat) and larynx (voice-box)

urea clearance test *see* **creatinine clearance test**

ureters two tubes (one from each from each kidney) which transport urine from the kidneys to the bladder

urethra the passage from the bladder through which urine is excreted, much longer in the male as it passses through the penis

urine retention inability to void urine

urogenital (UG) pertaining to the urinary and male reproductive systems

urology study/specialism of the functions of the urinary system

urticaria allergic skin eruption, eg in response to stinging nettles or penicillin

uterus the womb, a muscular sac lined with a mucous membrane, in which a fertilized embryo (fetus/baby) develops, usually for nine months before birth

vaccination injection of an antigen into a patient in order to stimulate artificial immunity to a disease (as the antigen stimulates production of antibodies to fight the disease-causing organism); *see* **antibody** and *cf* **immunization**, a different method of producing immunity

vagina muscular passage in females which leads outside the body from the uterus, used in conception and childbirth.

vaginitis inflammation of the vagina due to an infection. **vaginal swab** sample of fluid taken from vagina for laboratory testing for cancer and other diseases, or to investigate cause of discharge

varicella (chicken pox) mild, infectious viral disease, characterized by a rash of small blisters; common in childhood

varicose veins (VV) enlarged protruding veins, usually in the lower limbs, as a result of malfunctioning valves which may cause the blood to flow in reverse; sometimes causes un ulcer to form; may be operated upon to seal off affected veins

vas deferens in males, ducts situated on either side of the scrotum which secrete semen from the testes into the penis

vasectomy in males, surgical removal of part of the vas deferens usually for the purpose of sterilization, ie to prevent conception of a child; also sometimes performed to prevent infection following removal of the prostate gland

vein one of a network of vessels which return 'used' blood to the heart from around the body and also bring oxygenated blood back to the heart from the lungs for re-entry into the circulation, *cf* **arteries,** which carry blood *away* from the heart; veins branch into **venules** and then (tiny) capillaries. **pulmonary vein** vein which enters the heart containing oxygenated blood from the lungs. **superior vena cava/inferior vena cava** veins entering the top and bottom of the heart, which carry de-oxygenated (used) blood; Figure 5 show the blood's route through the heart

venereal disease (VD) a sexually-transmitted disease, ie any infectious disease whose primary means of spread is between sexual partners. **venereal disease reference laboratory (VDRL)** laboratory where blood samples are taken for diagnosis of syphilis

venogram (phlebogram) X-ray of a vein using a contrast medium

ventral pertaining to the frontal surface of the body, ie the face, chest, abdomen, etc

ventriculogram test to diagnose a cerebral (brain) tumour, involving the injection of air into a small hole in the skull

vertebrae the bones of the spine (back bone) which total 33, divided by type and function into five regions from the neck to base of the spine, called the **cervical**, **thoracic**, **lumbar** and **sacral** vertebrae and the **coccyx**; these give the back support and protect the spinal cord (nervous tissue running down to the 1st or 2nd lumbar vertebra) while allowing for a certain amount of flexibility in the back. **intervertebral disc** flat, rounded piece of cartilage which is situated between each vertebra

vertigo fear of heights, dizziness when high up

vesicle small hollow sac within the body or a skin blister

virus a type of micro-organism, made of protein and nucleic acid, many of which cause disease

vital capacity (of lungs) the maximum amount of air that can be expired following a deep breath; diminished capacity may indicate disease of the lungs

voluntary muscle a muscle which can be controlled at will, ie one that is attached to a bone and enables visible movement of the body; *cf* **involuntary muscle**

von Graefe's sign test to confirm hyperthyroidism, the excessive excretion of the hormone from the thyroid gland

vulva collective name for the external genitalia of the female

Wasserman reaction (WR) blood test to diagnose syphilis

Weber's test a hearing test, involving use of a tuning fork to distinguish between middle ear deafness and nerve deafness

well man clinic service offered by some general practices, of setting aside a particular time on a regular basis when men are invited to consult a doctor or nurse about risk factors for male-orientated diseases such as heart attacks and strokes (eg for measurement of blood pressure, cholesterol, weight, etc)

well woman clinic service offered by some general practices, of setting aside a particular time on a regular basis when women are invited to consult a doctor or nurse about matters specific to their sex, eg to ask for contraceptive advice or for a cervical screen or breast scan

white blood cells (WBC) (leucocytes) include various types of cells active in fighting infection, including lymphocytes (25%), formed in lymphoid tissue, which produce antibodies to give natural immunity to disease, and others which 'eat' bacteria; *see* Figure 1. **white blood count** laboratory test to check that the proportion of white cells in the blood is within the normal range; the number is raised in cases of leukaemia, pneumonia or appendicitis

whooping cough *see* pertussis

Widal reaction a blood test to diagnose typhoid or related conditions

windpipe *see* **trachea**

Wright's peak flow meter *see* **peak flow gauge**. Also used for diagnosing lung disease

X-ray *see* **radiography**

Appendix 1: Medical Word Structures

In clinical practice, the terms used to describe parts of the body and medical disorders are mainly of Latin or Greek origin. Those in common usage are generally known by English lay words. In order to learn the correct terminology, it is helpful to understand some of the language structures on which it is based.

Most medical terms consist of three parts:

prefix – root – suffix

The root forms the basis of the word; the prefix is a syllable added before the root to modify its meaning; and the suffix is a syllable added after the root to modify its meaning.

Prefixes indicate distinguishing characteristics such as position; eg *epi-* means on or above

Word roots indicate the disease process or the part of the body affected; eg *gastr* means stomach

Suffixes indicate the specific problem or context of reference; eg *-cele* means protrusion (**hernia**)

A combining vowel (usually 'o') links the root to another root or suffix. Thus the word **epigastrocele** means hernia of the upper stomach.

Word Roots

medical term	layman's term
aden	gland
ang	vessel (blood)
ankyl	crooked, looped
arter	artery
arthr/articul	joint
aud/aur	ear, hearing
bacill	bacteria
bios	life
blephar	eyelid
brach	arm
bronch	bronchus (tube leading into the lung)
bucc	cheek
carcin	cancer
card	heart
carp	wrist
caud	tail
cephal	head
cer	wax
cerebr	cerebrum (part of the brain)
cervic	neck
cheil	lip
cheir/chir	hand
chole	bile
cholecyst	gall-bladder
chondr	cartilage
clavic	clavicle
col	colon
colp	vagina
cort	covering
cost	rib
cran	cranium
cut	skin
cyst	bladder
cyte	cell

medical term	*layman's term*
dacry	tear duct
dactyl	finger, toe (digit)
dent/dont	tooth
derm	skin
dors	back
emesis	vomit
enter	intestine
erythr	red
faci	face, facies
fasci	band (fibrous)
galact	milk
gastr	stomach
genesis	birth
gingiv	gums
gloss	tongue
glyc	sugar
gnath	jaw
gravid	pregnant
gyn	woman
haem	blood
hallux	big toe
hepat	liver
hist	tissue
hydr	water
hyster	uterus (womb)
ile	ileum (part of intestine)
ili	ilium (part of hip bone)
kerat	horny, scaly/cornea
labia	lip
lacry	tear duct
lact	milk
lapar	abdomen
laryng	larynx
leuc	white
lingua	tongue
lip	fat
lith	stone
lymph	fluid (lymph)

medical term	layman's term
malar	cheek
mamm/mast	breast
medull	marrow/centre (of an organ)
melan	black
mensis	menstrual
metr	uterus
mnesis	memory
myc	fungus
myel	bone marrow/spinal cord
mys	muscle
nares	nose, nostrils
nas	nose
natus	birth
nephr	kidney
neur	nerve
ocul	eye
odont	tooth
omphalus	umbilicus
onych	finger-/toenail
oophor	ovary
ophthal	eye
or	mouth
orchidis/orchis	testes
orexia	appetite
os/oste	bone
oto	ear
ovar	ovary
ovi	egg
part	labour
ped/pod	foot
phagia	swallowing
pharyng	pharynx (throat)
phasia	speak, speech
phleb	vein
photo	light
phren	mind/diaphragm
physis	growth
pneumon	lung

medical term	*layman's term*
pnoea	breathing
pollex	thumb
proct	rectum
psyche	mind
pulmon	lung
pyel	pelvis (of the kidney)
pyo	pus
ren	kidney
rhin	nose
salping	ovarian tube
sarcoma	tumour, cancer
sclerosis	hardening
soma/somat	body
splanchno	internal organs
splen	spleen
spondyl	vertebra
squam	scaly
steth	chest
stoma	mouth
stric	narrowing
tars	foot
teno	tendon
thorac	thorax
thromb	clot (blood)
tox	poison
trache	trachea (windpipe)
trachel	neck
trich	hair
troph	nourish/feed
tussis	cough
tympan	eardrum
uro	urine
vas	vessel
ven	vein
vesic	bladder, sac
viscera	organ

Prefixes

prefix	meaning
a-/an-	absence
ab-	from/away from
acro-	extremity/point/end
ad-	to/near/towards
allo-	other
ambo-/amphi-	both
andro-	male
ante-	before/forward
anti-	against/opposite
atelo-	imperfect
auto-	self
bi-	two
brady-	slow
carcin-	cancerous
centi-	hundredth
circum-	around
co-/com-/con-	with/joined together/beside
contra-	against
cryo-	cold
crypto-	hidden
de-	down/from
deci-	tenth
dextr-	right (hand)
di-	two or disengage/separate
dia-	through/by means of
dis-	appart from/undo
dorsi-	back (of body)
dys-	difficult/painful
ec-/ecto-	out of/outer
endo-/ento-	within/inside
epi-	on/above
eu-	normal/favourable
ex-	out of
exo-/extra	outside

prefix	*meaning*
fibro-	fibrous
gen-	producing
hemi-	half
hetero-	different
homo-	same
hyper-	too much/excessive
hypo-	too little/beneath
iatro-	medicine
idio-/ipsi-	self
infra-	below/under
inter-	between
intra-/intro	into/in
iso-	same
laevo-	left (hand)
later-	side
macro-/mega-	large
mal-	abnormal/bad
medi-/meso-	middle
meta-	change
micro-	small
milli-	thousandth
mono-	single
multi-	many
myco-	fungal
nacro-	stupor
necro-	dead
neo-	new
non-	negative
norm-	normal
olig-	few
opthalm-	relating to the eyes
orth-	normal/straight
pachy-	thick
pan-	total
para-	beside
patho-	disease
per-	through/across
peri-	surrounding/around

prefix	*meaning*
pico-	small
poly-	many
post-	behind/after
pre-	in front of/before
proto-	first
pseud-	false
psych-	of the mind
quadr-	four
retro-	backward/back of
scler-	hard
semi-	half
sub-	under
super-	excess/above/beyond
supra-	superior/above
tachy-	rapid
tetr-	four
therm-	heat
trans-	through/across
tri	three
ultra-	beyond
uni-	one
ventri-	front (of body)
xero-	dry

Suffixes

Suffix	*meaning*
-aemia	blood condition
-aesthesia	feeling/sensation
-affine	affinity
-algia	pain
-ase	enzyme
-blast	embryonic form of a cell
-cele	swelling (containing fluid)
-centesis	puncture
-clast	cell with ability to destroy/break
-coccus	spherical bacterium
-cyst	sac of fluid
-cyte	cell
-desis	binding/fixation
-dynia	pain
-ectasis	dilation/expansion
-ectomy	excision
-ergia	movement
-genesis	forming/producing/condition of
-genic	origin
-gram	tracing
-graphy	recording
-gyria	rotation
-ia	disease
-iasis	condition/presence of (disease)
-ics	branch of medicine
-iform	resembling
-ist	practitioner
-itis	inflammation
-lysis	splitting/breaking down
-malacia	softening
-megaly	enlargement
-meter	measure
-mycosis	fungal
-oid	like/resembling

Suffix	*meaning*
-ol	alcohol
-ology	science or study of
-oma	tumour
-ose	sugar
-opia	eye/sight
-osis	disease/abnormal condition
-osmia	ability to smell
-ostomy	forming a mouth-like opening
-otomy	cutting into
-pathy	disease
-penia	lack of/deficiency
-pexy	fastening/fixation/suspension
-phasia	ability to speak
-philia	attraction
-phobia	fear of/repulsion
-plasty	construction/surgical correction/ artificial repair
-plegia	paralysis
-pnoea	breathing
-praxia	ability to (do something)
-rrhage	burst out
-rrhaphy	stitching/suturing
-rrhexis	burst out/rupture
-rrhoea	flow
-scopy	inspection/visualization
-somatic	of the body
-sonic	sound
-spasm	involuntary contraction
-stasis	lack of movement/stagnation
-taxia	arrangement/order
-tome	cutting
-topic	site
-tripsy	crushing
-trophy	nourishment/development

Appendix 2: Abbreviations and Symbols

Clinical Abbreviations

A & E	Accident and Emergency
A & W	alive and well
AB/ab	abortion
ACTH	adrenocorticotrophic hormone
AI	accidental injury
AID	artificial insemination donor
AIDS	acquired immune deficiency syndrome
AJ	ankle jerk
AN	anorexia nervosa/antenatal
ANA	antinuclear antibodies
ANS	autonomic nervous system
APH	antepartum haemorrhage
APM	anterior poliomyelitis
ARM	artificial rupture of membranes
Ba E	barium enema
Ba M	barium meal
BCC	basal cell carcinoma
BCG	Bacille-Calmette-Guérin (vaccine for TB)
BI	bony injury/bodily injury
BID	brought in dead
BMR	basal metabolic rate
BO	bowels open/body odour
BOA	born on arrival
BP	blood pressure
BSR	basal sedimentation rate
BW	birth weight
C	Celsius/centigrade
C/O	complains of
CAO	chronic airways obstruction

CAT	computerized axial tomography
CCF	congestive cardiac failure
CD	controlled drugs/cadaver donor
CDH	congenital dislocation of the hip
CF	cardiac failure
CHD	congenital heart disease
CK	creatine kinase
CNS	central nervous system
CSF	cerebrospinal fluid
CSSD	central sterile supply department
CSU	catheter specimen of urine
CT	coronary thrombosis/chemotherapy
CXR	chest X-ray
CVP	central venous pressure
CVS	cardiovascular system
D & C	dilatation and curettage (uterine)
D & V	diarrhoea and vomiting
DAT	differential agglutination test
DLE	disseminated lupus erythematous
DNA	did not attend/deoxyribonucleic acid
DOA	dead on arrival
DOB	date of birth
DS	disseminated sclerosis
DSA	digital subtraction angiogram
DT	delirium tremens
DTP	diphtheria, tetanus and pertussis (immunizations)
DU	duodenal ulcer/diagnosis undetermined
DVT	deep vein thrombosis
DXRT	deep X-ray therapy
ECG	electrocardiography
ECT	electroconvulsive therapy
EDC	expected date of confinement
EDD	expected date of delivery
EEG	electroencephalography
EMG	electromyogram
ENT	ear, nose and throat
ERCP	endoscopic retrograde cholangiopancreatography
ESN	educationally subnormal
ESR	erythrocyte sedimentation rate

EUA	examination under anaesthetic
EUS	external urethral sphincter
F	Fahrenheit/failure
FB	foreign body
FBC	full blood count
FBS	fasting blood sugar
FDIU	fetal death in utero
FHH	fetal heart heard
FHNH	fetal heart not heard
FSH	follicle stimulating hormone
Fx	fracture
GA	general anaesthetic
GCFT	gonorrhoea complement fixation test
GI	gastrointestinal
GG/gamma gl	gamma globulin
GH	growth hormone
GHRH	growth hormone release hormone
GOK	God only knows!
grav	gravid (pregnant)
GTT	glucose tolerance test
GU	gastric ulcer/genito-urinary
H & L	heart and lungs
Hb	haemoglobin
HbF	fetal haemoglobin
HCG	human chorionic gonadotrophin
HGG	human gamma globulin
Hib	Haemophilus influenzae type B
HIg	human immunoglobulin
HIV	human immunodefiency virus
HRT	hormone replacement therapy
HV	hallux valgus
HVS	high vaginal swab
IBS	irritable bowel syndrome
ICP	intracranial pressure
ICU	intensive care unit
IDK	internal derangement of the knee joint
Ig	immunoglobulin
IHD	ischaemic heart disease
IM	intramuscular
IOFP	intraocular foreign body
IQ	intelligence quotient

ISQ	in status quo
ITU	intensive therapy unit
IV	intravenous
IVP	intravenous pyelogram
IUCD	intrauterine contraceptive device
IUD	intrauterine death/intrauterine (contraceptive) device
JOD	juvenile onset diabetes
JV	jugular vein
JVP	jugular vein pulse/jugular venous pressure
KJ	knee jerk
KUB	kidneys, ureters and bladder
LA	local anaesthetic
LASER	light amplification by stimulated emission of radiation
LB	loose body
LBW	low birth weight
LE	lupus erythematosus/local excision
LFD	large for dates (fetus)
LFT	liver function tests
LG	lymph gland
LH	lutenizing hormone
LIF	left iliac fossa
LIH	left inguinal hernia
LLL	left lower lobe
LMP	last menstrual period
LOA	left occipito-anterior
LOL	left occipito-lateral
LOP	left occipito-posterior
LP	lumbar puncture
LRD	living related donor
LRTI	lower respiratory tract infection
LSCS	lower segment caesarian section
LVF	left ventricular failure
MAO	maximum acid output (gastric)/monoamine oxidase
MAOI	monoamine oxidase inhibitor
MCH	mean corpuscular haemoglobin
MCHC	mean corpuscular haemoglobin concentration
MCV	mean corpuscular volume

MI	myocardial infarction/mitral incompetence
MMR	measles, mumps and rubella (immunizations)
MPV	mean platelet volume
MRI	magnetic resonance imaging
MS	multiple sclerosis/mitral stenosis
MSSU/MSU	midstream specimen of urine
MVD	mitral valve disease
Mx	mastectomy
NAD	no abnormality demonstrated
NAI	non-accidental injury
NFS	no fracture seen/shown
NG	new growth
NGU	non-gonococcal urethritis
NMR	nuclear magnetic resonance
NND	neonatal death
NNMR	neonatal mortality rate
NPU	not passed urine
NSAIDS	non-steroid anti-inflammatory drugs
NSU	non-specific urethritis
NSV	non-specific vaginitis
NYD	not yet diagnosed
O_2	oxygen/both eyes
O & G	obstetrics and gynaecology
OA	osteoarthritis
OC	oral contraceptive
OGTT	oral glucose tolerance test
OP	out-patient
OPD	out-patient department
OPV	oral poliomyelitis vaccine
OT	occupational therapy
PA	pernicious anaemia
PBI	protein bound iodine
PBU	premature baby unit
PCV	packed cell volume
PE	plasma exchange/pulmonary embolism
PEFR	peak expiratory flow rate
PG	prostaglandins
PG/pg	pregnant
PID	prolapsed intervertebral disc/pelvic inflammatory disease
PIFR	peak inspiratory flow rate

PKU	phenylketonuria
PM	pacemaker/post-mortem
PMA	progressive muscular atrophy
PMB	post-menopausal bleeding
PMH	post-menopausal haemorrhage/past medical history
PMS	pre-menstrual syndrome
PMT	pre-menstrual tension
PNM	perinatal mortality
PO	per os (by mouth)
POP	plaster of Paris
PPH	post-partum haemorrhage
PR/pr	per rectum
PROM	premature rupture of membranes
PU	peptic ulcer/passed urine
PUO	pyrexia of unknown origin
PV	per vagina
RA	rheumatoid arthritis
RAO	right anterior oblique
RB	recurrent bleed
RBC	red blood cells
RDS	respiratory distress syndrome
RE	rectal examination
Rh	rhesus factor
RIF	right iliac fossa
RIH	right inguinal hernia
RL shunt	right–left shunt
RLL	right lower lobe
RNA	ribonucleic acid
ROA	right occipito-anterior
ROM	range of movements/rupture of membranes
ROP	right occipito-posterior
ROT	right occipito-transverse
RPR	rapid plasma reagin
RS	respiratory system
RT	radiotherapy
RTA	road traffic accident
RU	rodent ulcer
RUL	right upper lobe
RV	residual volume

S_1, S_2, S_3, S_4	1st, 2nd, 3rd and 4th heart sounds
SAB	systolic arterial blood pressure
SB	stillbirth/Stanford-Binet (intelligence) tests
SCAN	suspected child abuse or neglect
SCBU	special care baby unit
SCC	squamous cell carcinoma
SDAT	senile dementia Alzheimer's type
SIDS	sudden infant death syndrome
SLE	systemic lupus erythematosus
SMR	submucous resection of nasal septum
SOB	shortness of breath
SOL	space occupying lesion
SPAM	scanning photo-acoustic microscopy
STD	sexually transmitted disease
STOP	suction termination of pregnancy
STYCAR	Sheridan tests for young children and retards
SUD	sudden unexpected death
T & A	tonsils and adenoids
TAB	typhoid A and B (vaccines)
TB	tubercle bacillus
TCA	tricyclic antidepressant/to come again
TCI	to come in
TFT	thyroid function tests
THA	total hip arthroplasty
THR	total hip replacement
TJR	total joint replacement
TKR	total knee replacement
TL	tubal ligation
TLC	tender loving care
TLE	temporal lobe epilepsy
TMJ	temporomandibular joint
TOP	termination of pregnancy
TPHA	treponema pallidum haemoglutination
TPN	total parenteral nutrition
TPR	temperature, pulse and respiration
TSSU	theatre sterile supply unit
TUR	transurethral resection (of prostate)
TX	transplant
UC	ulcerative colitis
UG	urogenital

URTI	upper respiratory tract infection
UTI	urinary tract infection
US	ultrasound
UVR	ultraviolet rays
V	volume of tidal air
VD	venereal disease
VDRL	venereal disease reference laboratory
VE	vaginal examination
VSD	ventricular septal defect
VV	varicose veins
Vx	vertex (of fetus)
WBC	white blood cells
WR	Wassermann reaction
XR	X-ray

Other Medical Abbreviations (including job titles, organizations and non-clinical terms)

AHCPA*	Association of Health Centres and Practice Administrators
AMSPAR*	Association of Medical Secretaries, Practice Administrators and Receptionists
BAMM	British Association of Medical Managers
BMA*	British Medical Association
BMJ	British Medical Journal
BNF	British National Formulary
BP	British Pharmacopoeia
BPC	British Pharmaceutical Codex
BRCS	British Red Cross Society
CHC	Community Health Council
CMB	Central Midwives Board
CME	continuing medical education
CNO	Chief Nursing Officer
DDA	Dangerous Drugs Act
DHA	District Health Authority
DN	district nurse
DoH	Department of Health
DSS	Department of Social Security
FHSA	Family Health Services Authority
FPA	Family Planning Association
GDP	general dental practitioner
GMC*	General Medical Council
GMSC	General Medical Services Committee
GMP	general medical practitioner
GP	general practitioner
HV	health visitor
IHSM*	Institute of Health Services Management
IMA	independent medical adviser
LMC	Local Medical Committee
MAAG	Medical Audit Advisory Group
MDU	Medical Defence Union

* address supplied on page 116.

MIMS	Monthly Index of Medical Specialties
MPS	Medical Protection Society
MSW	medical social worker
NAHAT*	National Association of Health Authorities and Trusts
NBTS	National Blood Transfusion Service
NHS	National Health Service
OT	occupational therapist
PACT	prescribing analyses and costs
PGEA	postgraduate education allowance
QALY	quality adjusted life year
RCGP*	Royal College of General Practitioners
RCN	Royal College of Nursing
RGN	Registered General Nurse
RHA	Regional Health Authority
RN	Registered Nurse
SEN	State Enrolled Nurse
SHO	Senior House Officer
SI	Systeme Internationale (units)
SRN	State Registered Nurse
TQM	total quality management
UKCC	United Kingdom Council for Nursing, Midwifery and Health Visiting
WHO	World Health Organization

* **address supplied on page 117.**

Abbreviations used in prescribing

abbreviation	Latin term (if applicable)	meaning
aa	ana	of each amount
ac	ante cibum	before meals
alt die	alt die	alternate days
alt noct	alt nocte	alternate nights
aq ad	aqua ad	water as desired
aurist	auristillae	ear drops
bid/bd	bis in die	twice daily
c	cum	with
caps	capsules	capsules
cc		cubic cm
collut	collutores	mouth wash
collyr	collyria	eye lotion
consp	conspersi	dusting powder
crem	cremore	cream
dil		dilute
elix		elixir
emuls		emulsion
ex aq	ex aqua	in water
ext		extract
garg		gargle
gutt	guttae	eye drops
hm	hac mane	this morning
hd	hora dicubitus	at bedtime
hn	hac nocte	tonight
hs	hora somni	at bedtime
im		intramuscular
inj		injection
iv		intravenous
lin		linament
linct		linctus
liqu	liquore	solution
lot		lotion
m et n	mane et nocte	morning and night
m et sign	misce et signa	mix and label
mane	mane	in the morning

abbreviation	*Latin term* (if applicable)	*meaning*
mdu	more dicta utendus	as previously directed
mist	mistura	mixture
mitte	mitte	to send
narist	naristillae	nasal drops
nocte	nocte	at night
oc	occulentae	eye ointment
od	omni die	once daily
om	omni mane	every morning
on	omni nocte	every night
pa	parti affectae	affected part
pc	post cibum	after meals
pess		pessary
pig	pigmentae	paint
prn	pro re nata	whenever necessary
pulv	pulvere	powder
qds/qid	quater die sumendum/quater in die	four times daily
qq	quaque	every
qqh	quarta quaque hora	every fourth hour
qs	quantum sufficit	as much as required
R	recipe	take (prescription)
rep	repititur	repeat
S	semis	a half
sig	signa	label
sos	si opus sit	if necessary
SS	semi-semis	a quarter
stat	statim	immediately
suppos		suppository
syr		syrup
tabs		tablets
tds/tid	ter die sumendum/ ter in die	three times daily
troch	trochiisci	lozenges
tuss urg	tussi urgenti	when cough is troublesome
ung	unguenta	ointment
vap	vapore	inhalation

Medical Symbols

♂	male
♀	female
#	fracture
△	diagnosis
℞	recipe (for prescription, 'take thou')
+ve	positive
−ve	negative
/c	with
/s	without
1/7	one day (per week)
3/7	three days (per week)
1/52	one week
1/12	one month

Appendix 3: Immunization Schedules

Recommended Immunizations for Children

The schedule below is currently recommended by the Department of Health.

Age	Disease	Method
at birth (high risk infants only)	tuberculosis hepatitis B	injection (BCG) injection
4 weeks (high risk infants only)	hepatitis B	injection
2 months	diphtheria, tetanus, pertussis Haemophilus influenza type B (Hib) polio	one injection (DTP) injection by mouth (OPV)
3 months	diphtheria, tetanus pertussis Haemophilus influenza type B (Hib) polio	one injection (DTP) injection by mouth (OPV)
4 months	diphtheria, tetanus pertussis Haemophilus influenza type B polio	one injection (DTP) injection by mouth (OPV)

Age	Disease	Method
12–15 months (usually 14)	measles, mumps, rubella	one injection (MMR)
4–5 years	diphtheria ⎫ tetanus ⎬ polio ⎭	booster injections booster by mouth (OPV)
10–14 years (girls only)	rubella	one injection
13 years	tuberculosis	one injection (BCG)
15–19 years	polio	booster by mouth (OPV)
16–18 years (school leavers)	tetanus	one injection

Recommended Immunizations for Adults

Disease	Frequency	Method
tetanus toxoid	booster every 10 years	one injection, or 3 at monthly intervals for those previously unvaccinated
polio	booster every 10 years until age 40	by mouth (OPV)

For at-risk groups:

Disease	Frequency	Method
influenza	annually (especially for the elderly)	injection
hepatitis B	booster every 3–5 years	injection (in 1st instance, 3 over 6 months, followed by a blood test)

Travellers to hot climates and developing countries should be given immunizations and antimalarial advice according to the up-to-date recommendations in the *Pulse* and *Mims* charts published monthly, and the patient's previous immunization status.

Appendix 4: The Structure of the National Health Service

```
                        ┌──────┐
                        │ DoH  │
                        └──────┘
```

Number: 1 each for England, Scotland, Wales and Northern Ireland.
Composition: for whole of UK, Secretary of State for Health, Minister of State for Health, junior ministers, >5000 civil servants including the Permanent Secretary, CMO (one for each DoH) and the Chief Executive of the NHS Management Executive.
Role: Policy Board sets strategies. Composed from businessmen, NHS personnel, Government officials and health ministers. Chaired by the Secretary of State.
Role: NHS Management Executive has operational responsibility. Comprises businessmen and civil servants. Chaired by the Chief Executive.
The DoH issues policy statements (White Papers); advises health authorities; funds, monitors and holds to account RHAs.

```
  ┌──────┐        ┌──────┐        ┌────────────┐
  │ RHAs │        │ SHAs │        │ NHS Trusts │
  └──────┘        └──────┘        └────────────┘
```

Number: 17 in UK (14 in England).
Composition: 5 members appointed by Secretary of State, and up to 5 executive members.
Role: plan and allocate resources (including building projects); implement Government reforms, oversee DHAs; regulate purchaser-provider transactions.

Role: administer special activities.
Include: HEA, MHAC, NHSTA, SHSA.

Composition: up to 5 members appointed by RHA/ Secretary of State, and up to 5 executive members.
Role: self-governing NHS hospitals.

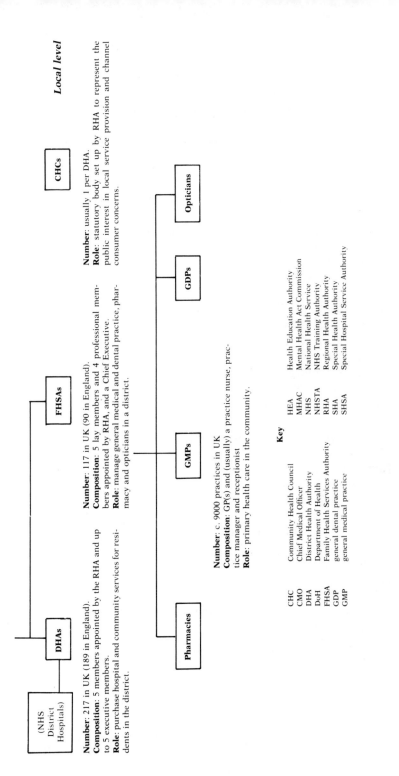

Local level

(NHS District Hospitals)

DHAs

FHSAs

CHCs

Pharmacies — **GMPs** — **GDPs** — **Opticians**

DHAs
Number: 217 in UK (189 in England).
Composition: 5 members appointed by the RHA and up to 5 executive members.
Role: purchase hospital and community services for residents in the district.

FHSAs
Number: 117 in UK (90 in England).
Composition: 5 lay members and 4 professional members appointed by RHA, and a Chief Executive.
Role: manage general medical and dental practice, pharmacy and opticians in a district.

CHCs
Number: usually 1 per DHA.
Role: statutory body set up by RHA to represent the public interest in local service provision and channel consumer concerns.

GMPs
Number: c. 9000 practices in UK
Composition: GP(s) and (usually) a practice nurse, practice manager and receptionist
Role: primary health care in the community.

Key

CHC	Community Health Council	HEA	Health Education Authority
CMO	Chief Medical Officer	MHAC	Mental Health Act Commission
DHA	District Health Authority	NHS	National Health Service
DoH	Department of Health	NHSTA	NHS Training Authority
FHSA	Family Health Services Authority	RHA	Regional Health Authority
GDP	general dental practice	SHA	Special Health Authority
GMP	general medical practice	SHSA	Special Hospital Service Authority

Appendix 5: Useful Addresses

Association of Health Centres and Practice Administrators (AHCPA)
c/o Royal College of General Practitioners
14 Princes Gate
London SW7 1PU
Tel: 071 581 3232

Association of Medical Secretaries, Practice Administrators and Receptionists (AMSPAR)
Room 70, Block A
Tavistock House North
Tavistock Square
London WC1H 9LN
Tel: 071 387 600

British Medical Association (BMA)
BMA House
Tavistock Square
London WC1H 9JP
Tel: 071 387 4499

General Medical Council (GMC)
44 Hallam Street
London W1
Tel: 071 580 7642

Institute of Health Services Management (IHSM)
75 Portland Place
London W1N 4AN
Tel: 071 580 5041

National Association of Health Authorities and Trusts (NAHAT)
Birmingham Research Park
Vincent Drive
Birmingham B15 2SQ
Tel: 021 471 4444

Royal College of General Practitioners (RCGP)
14 Princes Gate
London SW7 1PU
Tel: 071 581 3232